Sport and Oral Health

Siobhan C. Budd • Jean-Christophe Egea

Sport and Oral Health

A Concise Guide

Springer

Siobhan C. Budd
Faculty of Dental Surgery
University of Montpellier
Montpellier
France

Jean-Christophe Egea
Faculty of Dental Surgery
University of Montpellier
Montpellier
France

ISBN 978-3-319-85150-1 ISBN 978-3-319-53423-7 (eBook)
DOI 10.1007/978-3-319-53423-7

Printed on acid-free paper

This Springer imprint is published by Springer Nature
The registered company is Springer International Publishing AG
The registered company address is: Gewerbestrasse 11, 6330 Cham, Switzerland

Jules, Antoine and Anne-Sophie

Preface

Sport is integral to contemporary society. It enriches social and cultural relations, induces economic prosperity and improves both the physical and psychological wellbeing of those taking part.

Despite the irrefutable health benefits of regular exercise, the implications for oral health have been largely overlooked. Of interest to the sporting population, dental practitioners and health professionals alike, this guide aims to heighten awareness and promote a deeper understanding of the interrelationship between sporting performance and oral health.

The first part of this guide enters the multifaceted world of training and performance. An understanding of the physiological and psychological demands athletes face permits an identification of the oral health risks linked to exercise.

The second section classifies and explains each of these specific sports-related risks, ranging from hyposalivation, modified eating habits, traumatology and immunological modifications to even the lack of prioritisation of dental care amongst the sporting population.

This is followed by a comprehensive clinical guide to common periodontal and dental consequences and how problems such as malocclusion, infection and dental pain can interfere with sporting performance.

To conclude, the key elements of personal and professional dental management are addressed, including the need for a collaboration between a wide range of specialists. These include specific preventative strategies and therapeutic solutions which promote optimal oral health and help athletes reach peak performance.

Montpellier, France

Siobhan C. Budd
Jean-Christophe Egea

Acknowledgements

Dr. Christel Dessalces Olenisac
Dr. Matthieu Renaud
Temps Course, Montpellier
Faculté d'Odontologie, Université de Montpellier, France.

Contents

Abbreviations

AAS	Anabolic androgenic steroids
AFLD	Association Française de Lutte contre le Dopage
BEWE	Basic erosive wear examination
BMI	Body mass index
CNS	Central nervous system
EPO	Erythropoietin
HIIT	High-intensity interval training
ICR	Individual caries risk
KCal	Kilocalorie
KJ	Kilojoule
MET	Metabolic equivalent value
pH	Potential of hydrogen
TMJ	Temporomandibular joint
VAS	Visual analogue scale
Vmart	Maximal anaerobic velocity
VO_2 MAX	Maximal oxygen uptake
vVO_2	Maximal velocity at maximal oxygen uptake
VRS	Verbal rating scale

Part I

Sport, Athletes and Training

An understanding of sport, athletes and their training methods gives an invaluable insight into the rise of sports-related oral health risks.

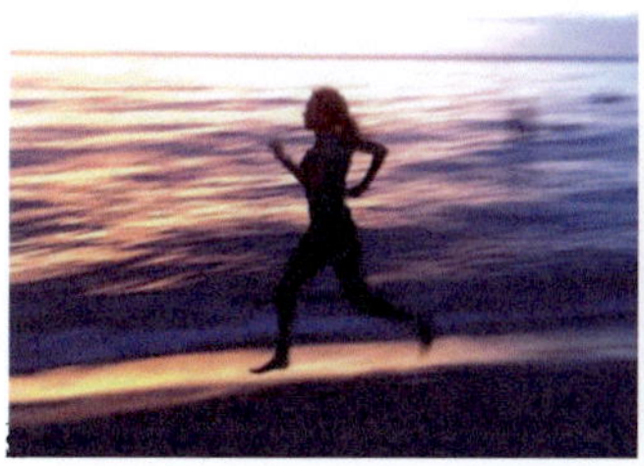
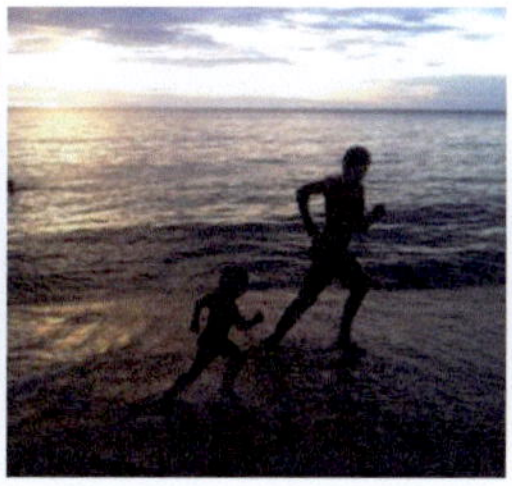
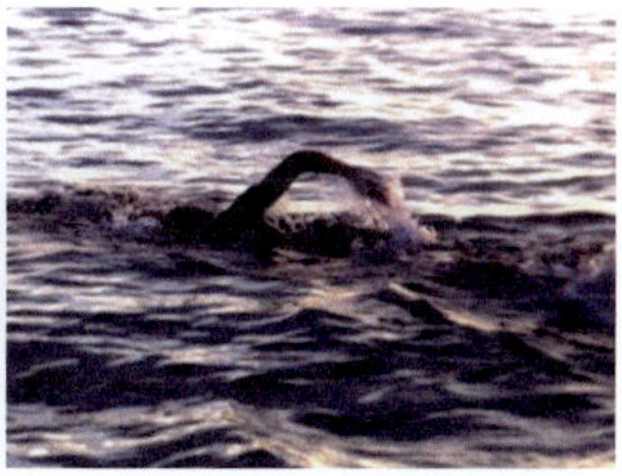

The Evolution of Sport in Society 1

1.1 Introduction

Sport is everywhere. Whether as a participant or a spectator, people of different ages, socio-economic standing, cultures and countries are involved in sport. Sport has become an influential financial industry, a favourite recreational pastime and an essential element of good health. But how did such an important element of modern society evolve?

Evidence of sport in society dates back thousands of years. Initially as local games and competitions, it was a male pastime. Major organised sporting events, such as the ever popular Olympic Games, commenced in Greece in 776 BC and are still enjoyed in the twenty-first century.

Colonisation spread the notion of sport across the continents, and the rise of mass media instigated the concept of professional sport during the twentieth century. The gender gap has narrowed in recent decades, partially due to the drive for women's rights.

Currently, American civilians enjoy a wide range of sporting activities, with baseball, basketball and American football forming part of their national identity. Sport is universal.

1.2 The First Traces of Sport

Evidence of competitive sport in society dates back hundreds of centuries. Indeed, the earliest indications of sport are the cave paintings dating back around 17,300 years found in France, showing wrestling and sprinting (Capelo 2010). Several thousand years later, stone slabs from the Sumerian civilization, around 3000 BC, show pairs wrestling (Crawford 2004). Equally, monuments to the Pharaohs show Egyptians enjoying several sports including athletics and ball games around 2000 BC (Fig. 1.1) (Hamblin 2006).

S.C. Budd, J.-C. Egea, *Sport and Oral Health*, DOI 10.1007/978-3-319-53423-7_1

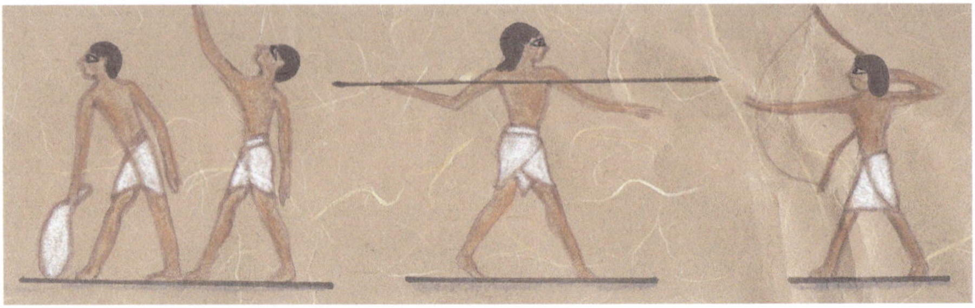

Fig. 1.1 Sports enjoyed in ancient Egypt: weightlifting, athletics and archery

The popularity of ball games in very different civilisations continued into more modern historical times. During the European Middle Ages, the Italian aristocracy favoured ball games, and English villages would compete against each other in often rough and violent games. Ball games are still integral to current day sport.

1.3 The Emergence of the Olympics

The first ever recorded Olympic Games took place in Greece in 776 BC, where running was the only event – a great contrast to the recent Rio de Janeiro Olympics 2016, where 41 different sports were represented (Official Site of the Olympic Games 2016). The games took place every 4 years, with a gradual inclusion of additional events, such as jumping and throwing events in later games. This sequence of the games ended in 393 AD.

Seventeen centuries later, Olympiads in Britain and France are believed to be the forerunners of the modern Olympic Games. Reinstated in Greece in 1859, play recommenced and would occur every 4 years up until the present day (Arvin-Bérod 1996).

1.4 Men and Women in Sport

In most premodern societies, families only encouraged fathers and sons to compete in sports – a strictly male activity. Nowadays, though women are still outnumbered, the gender gap has narrowed considerably (NFHS Report 2015).

The twentieth century witnessed a major increase in women's participation partly related to the drive for more women's rights. In the USA, female students' participation in sports was significantly boosted by the Title IX Act in 1972 (Federal Register 1979) which ensured equal opportunity for women to get involved in sport at all levels. This progression in equality is reflected in the prominence of female teams in the North American interscholastic and intercollegiate landscape and in private sports clubs across the globe.

1.5 Global Expansion: Modern-Day Sport

In the early nineteenth and twentieth centuries, North America and Western Europe predominantly defined the rules and format of modern events in athletics and other sports. It was then the historical phenomenon of colonisation that instigated the spread of both team and individual sports throughout the world (The British Empire and post-colonial sports: development of modern sports 2016).

The advent of global communication and mass media since the 1960s has encouraged the increase in professional sport. Let us take football (soccer) as an example. Most countries host league games at various levels of competence and participate in a variety of international matches. The *Fédération Internationale de Football Association* (FIFA) estimated that at the turn of the twenty-first century, there were approximately 250 million football players and over 1.3 billion people 'interested' in football. In 2010, for example, a combined television audience of more than *26 billion* watched football's premier tournament, the World Cup.

1.5.1 Modern-Day American Sport

The most popular sports currently played in the USA are baseball, basketball and American football.

Baseball, despite its global influence and the growing popularity in Asian and Latin American leagues, is the sport that Americans still recognise as their 'national pastime'. The game has long been woven into the fabric of American life and identity.

Basketball's popularity exploded at all levels towards the end of the twentieth century, thanks to increased exposure on television. It quickly moved to the forefront of the American sporting scene, alongside traditional leaders such as baseball and football. Four areas of the game developed during this period: US high school and college basketball, professional basketball, women's basketball and international basketball. All 50 states now conduct annual statewide tournaments.

American football originally evolved from soccer and rugby football at the elite American universities and now attracts the greatest number of spectators of the three major American team sports. In recent times, it has been exported to Europe where it has achieved a degree of international popularity (The History of Sports in the United States 2016).

The evolution of sport and its place in contemporary society has been greatly dependent on cultural preferences, global integration and more recently the role of international media. The twenty-first century boasts global participation in hundreds of sports. Adapted to men, women and children of all ages and ability, sport is for everyone (Fig. 1.2).

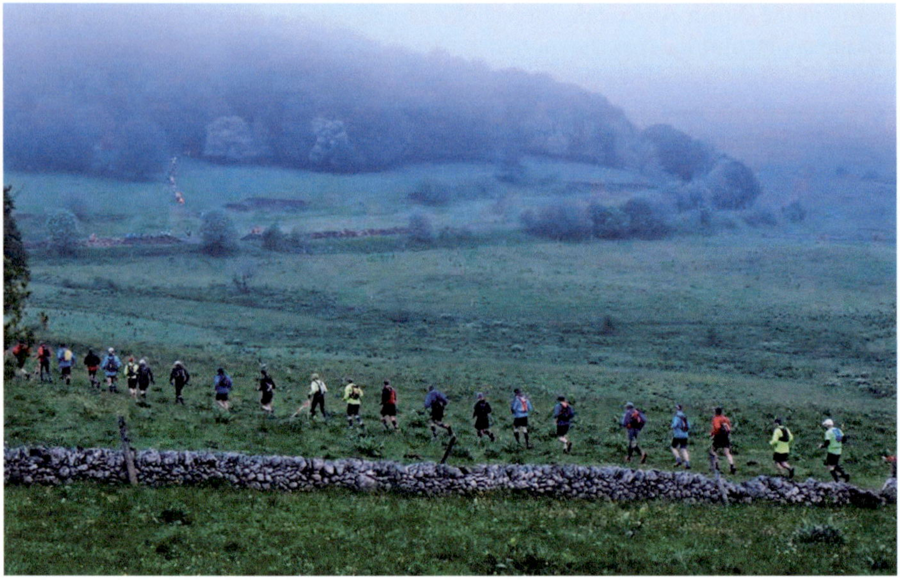

Fig. 1.2 Sport is for everyone

References

Arvin-Bérod A (1996) Les enfants d'Olympie. CERF, Paris

Capelo H (2010) Symbols from the Sky: heavenly messages from the depths of prehistory may be encoded on the walls of caves throughout Europe. Seed Magazine

Crawford H (2004) Sumer and the Sumerians. Cambridge: Cambridge University Press, p 247

Federal Register (1979) A policy interpretation: Title IX and Intercollegiate Athletics. 44;239:71413–71423

Hamblin WJ (2006) Warfare in the Ancient Near East to 1600BC. Routledge, Utah

NFHS Report (2015) https://nfhs.org/articles/high school sports participation increases for 26th consecutive year. Accessed 23 Aug 2016

Official Site of the Olympic Games (2016) Summer sports. https://www.olympic.org. Accessed 2 Sept 2016

The British Empire and post-colonial sports: development of modern sports. https://en.wikipedia.org/wiki. Accessed 28 Aug 2016

The History of Sports in the United States. http://www.topendsports.com/world/countries/usa.htm. Accessed 19 Aug 2016

The Popularity and Benefits of Sport and Exercise: Implications in Dentistry

2

2.1 Introduction

A phenomenal increase in male and female participation has been globally witnessed since the 1970s. This wave of popularity has been largely due to the combination of a fast-paced modern lifestyle and an increased awareness of the importance of health. Many individuals now turn to sport and exercise to accomplish and maintain both physical and mental fitness. For example, sports such as running, cycling and swimming are an effective way to stay in shape and relieve stress. Let us take the example of high-intensity interval training (HIIT). Based on hard efforts over very short time periods, these tough sessions are easily adaptable to different sports, time constraints and the capacity of the individual doing them – a very efficient way of developing all elements of fitness.

People of *all ages* are therefore currently involved in sport, representing an increased number of active patients in dental surgeries. Recent studies have revealed numerous potential oral health risk factors connected to sport. It is time to increase awareness of dental practitioners, health professionals and indeed athletes in order to prevent these complications.

2.2 Implications for the Dental Care Team

The number of dental patients involved in sport is therefore increasing. However, despite the pursuit of optimal physical and mental health, oral health is often undervalued. In comparison to their sedentary counterparts, people who regularly exercise are predisposed to a number of potential oral health risk factors (Frese et al. 2014). These are linked to training methods, the nutritional demands of physical exercise and hyposalivation during sporting effort. Up until recent times, little emphasis has been placed upon the link between oral health and sport, though several pertinent studies have concentrated on *elite athletes* and oral repercussions. The dental surgeon must be aware that active patients of all abilities are

S.C. Budd, J.-C. Egea, *Sport and Oral Health*, DOI 10.1007/978-3-319-53423-7_2

susceptible to risks aggravating certain hard and soft tissue lesions. They must appreciate the interaction between dental problems and sporting performance and be able to provide suitable treatment plans adapted to their individual needs. In collaboration with other health professionals, the dentist forms part of a team that helps the sporting patient achieve their potential and maximise their overall health and wellbeing.

2.3 Understanding Participation: The Benefits of Sport and Exercise

Physiologically speaking, the benefits of regular exercise are undeniable. The numerous advantages include a reduced risk of myocardial infarction and the prevention of certain malignancies, diabetes and high blood pressure. Sport promotes longevity of life, retards the onset of dementia and is considered an antidepressant (Sharma et al. 2015). Aerobic forms of exercise that endure 20 to 40 minutes improve morale over several hours (Raglin 1990).

According to a recent nationwide poll of American adults, the benefits of sport perceived by the public were improved mental and physical health, reduced stress and improved perception of their appearance (Fig. 2.1). Furthermore, their professional and social lives flourished (NPR 2015).

Such results were closely correlated to their reasons for participating in sport and exercise (Fig. 2.2). Whether participating in certain sports or partaking in different exercises, the main reasons were for personal enjoyment and satisfaction and to optimise health and wellbeing.

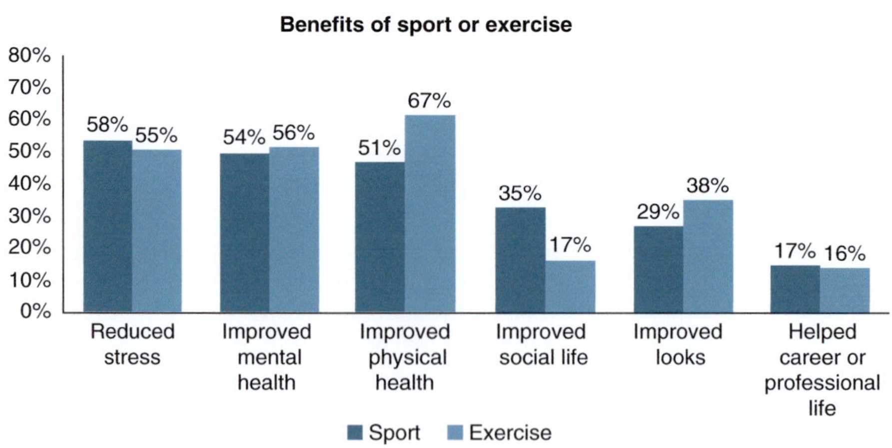

Fig. 2.1 The benefits of sport and exercise

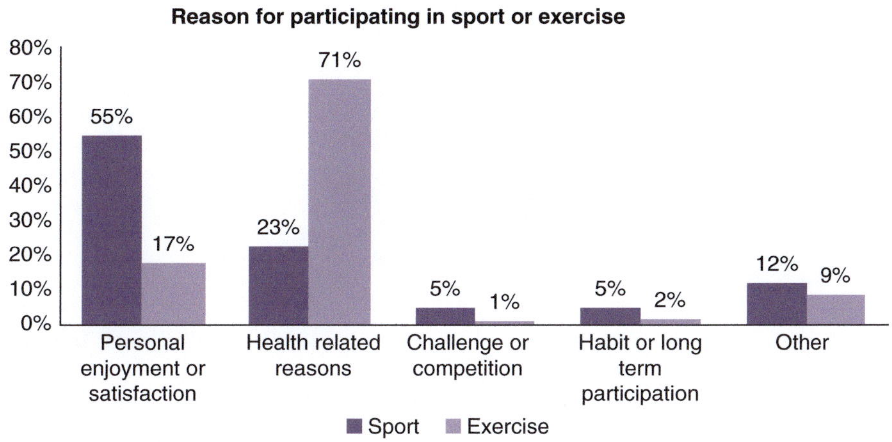

Fig. 2.2 The reasons for participating in sport and exercise

2.4 Participation in Sport and Exercise: A Few Statistics

Across the Atlantic, the Eurobarometer survey of all 28 European Union member states on sport and physical activity (European Commission 2004), showed similar socio-demographic trends to those from the USA. However, it revealed a considerable variation in the numbers participating in sport across the member states. Northern European countries such as Sweden were the most active, with 70% of the population engaged in weekly exercise. Equally, French national statistics revealed that in the last few years, two-thirds of the French population participated in sporting activity every week. Half of those who did regular activity were affiliated to sporting federations. Endurance sports clubs proved to be the most popular to join (Ministère des Droits 2014).

To illustrate the popularity of sport and exercise, we need only to look at the renowned road running classical endurance event – the marathon (42.195 km). It celebrates huge success across the world, inviting runners of all abilities to challenge this gruelling feat. Nearly 50,000 people participated in the New York Marathon in 2016, and the Paris marathon attracted 43,317 competitors and London approximately 38,000. Such high levels of participation in just one event give an insight into just how many individuals could be affected by sports-related dental problems.

2.5 The Participation of Children in Sport

Children participating in sport from an early age equally reap an array of benefits. Like adults, their physical and mental health is optimised, as are the emotional, social and educational sides of their development. According to parents of American children, again investigated by the 2015 national poll, the perceived benefits of their participation in sport also included development of discipline and dedication, team

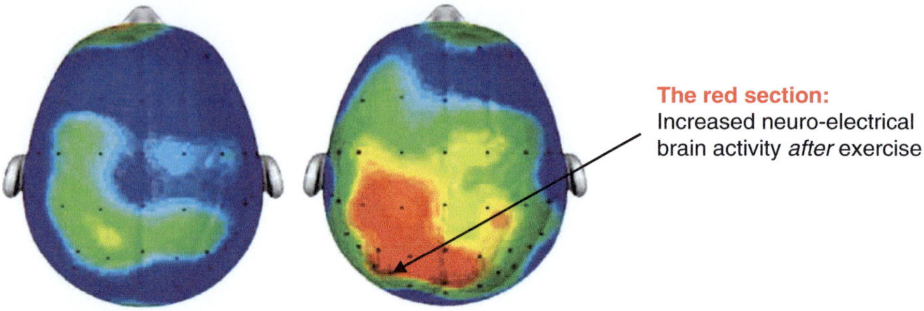

Fig. 2.3 Brain activity of children before and after exercise: a 20 minute walk (Source: Dr Chuck Hillman, University of Illinois)

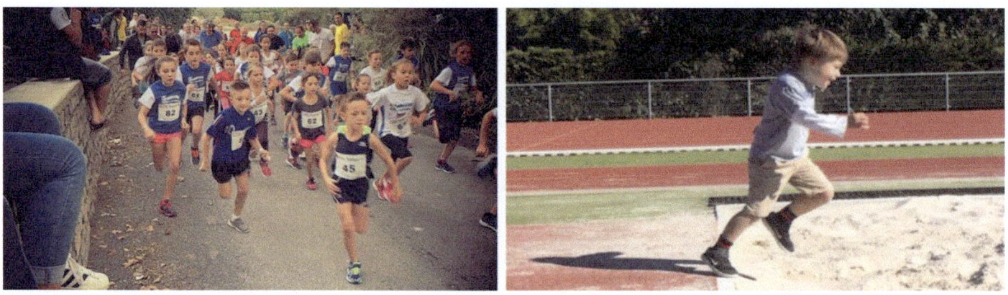

Fig. 2.4 Children in sport

cohesion, improved social life and skills positively contributing to both further education and careers (NPR 2015). Studies show that adolescents engaged in sporting activities are eight times as likely to continue the sport into adulthood (Perkins 2004).

An interesting study by Chuck Hillman, of the University of Illinois, investigated the cerebral neuroelectrical activity of 20 school children (Hillman 2009). A first MRI scan was taken after 20 min of sitting quietly and a second after a 20 minute walk (Fig. 2.3). Results revealed greater brain activity after physical exercise. This confirms that the benefits of sport and exercise, for both children and adults, stretch far beyond the initial obvious physical gains.

Finally, encouraging greater participation of children and adolescents in sport (Fig. 2.4) is also a key element of the battle against the global rise of obesity (Aspen Institute 2015). In the USA, the number of participants in high school sports increased for the 26th consecutive year in 2014–2015 – topping the 7.8 million mark for the first time (National Federation of State High School Federations).

2.6 Disabled Athletes in Sport

Increasing numbers of people with disabilities have been helped and encouraged to participate in sporting activities across many countries. This positive trend has been reinforced by the 2008 United Nations Convention on the Rights of Persons with Disabilities (Article 30):

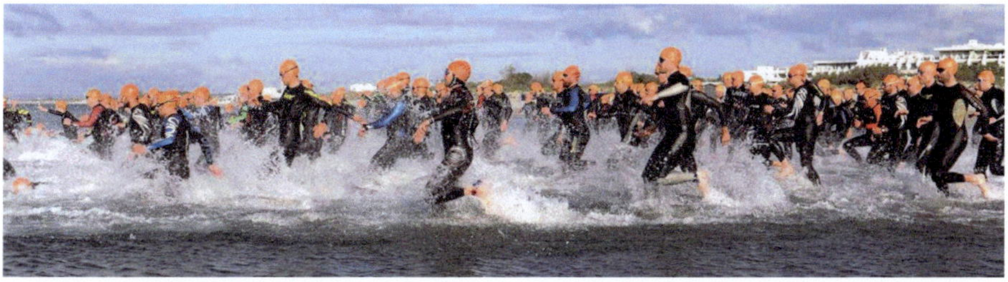

Fig. 2.5 The popularity of sport

> People with disabilities have the right to take part in cultural life on an equal basis with others, including access to cultural materials, performances and services, and to recreational, leisure and sporting activities.

The expanding numbers of Paralympians reflect the changing motivation and inclusion in sporting activities. In the 1960 Rome Olympics, 23 countries were represented by 400 athletes. In London 2012, over 4000 athletes from 164 countries took part (Australian Paralympics Committee 2016).

The sporting world is embracing more and more people (Fig. 2.5).

References

Australian Paralympic Committee. Paralympic education programme – history of the games. https://www.paralympiceducation.org.au. Accessed 19 July 2016

European Commission (2004) Special eurobarometer 412. Sport and physical activity. http://ec.europa.eu/health/sites/health/files/nutrition_physical_activity/docs/ebs_412_en.pdf. Accessed 16 Dec 2016

Frese CF, Frese S, Kuhlmann D, Saure D, Reljic HJ, Staehle HJ, Wolff D et al (2014) Effect of endurance training on dental erosion, caries, and saliva. Scand J Med Sci Sports. https://www.ncbi.nlm.nih.gov/pubmed/24917276. Accessed 15 Feb 2016

Hillman CH et al (2009) The effect of acute treadmill walking on cognitive control and academic achievement in preadolescent children. Neuroscience 159:1044–1055

Ministère de Droits Des Femmes, De la Ville, De la Jeunesse et Des Sports. Les chiffres clés du sport (2014) https://www.sports.gouv.fr/IMG/pdf. Accessed Nov 2015

NPR, Robert Johnson Foundation, Harvard T.H. Chan School of Public Health. Sport and Health in America. (2015) http://media.npr.org/documents/2015/june/sportsandhealthpoll.pdf. Accessed 23 Aug 2016

Perkins DF, Jocobs JE, Barber BL, Eccles JS (2004) Childhood and adolescent sports participation as predicators of participation in sports and physical fitness activities during young adulthood. Youth Soc 35(4):495–520. doi:10.1177/0044118X03261619

Raglin JS (1990) Exercise and mental health. Beneficial and detrimental effects. Sports med (Auckl, NZ) 6:323–329

Sharma S, Merghani A, Mont L (2015) Exercise and the heart: the good, the bad, and the ugly. Eur Heart J 36(23):1445–1453

The Aspen Institute. Facts: sports activity and children – reimaging youth sports in America (2015) http://www.aspenprojectplay.org/the-facts. Accessed 05 Sep 2016

Specifics of Physical Sports and Athletes: Different Types of Athletic Patients

3

3.1 Introduction

Sport improves the physiological and psychological wellbeing of participants. It also promotes social and cultural cohesion and is characterised by an element of competition, regardless of the level of play.

Focus is upon physical sports, one of several categories of sport that are internationally recognised. It may be distinguished from physical activity and exercise by the imposition of certain regulations governing play. However, all are closely interrelated. Equally, athletes who participate in sports are individuals who *compete*, train regularly and abide by these rules of conduct.

The physiological demands of different sports vary. At one extreme, endurance sports rely upon aerobic development and are favoured by athletes of ectomorphic morphology. Inversely, explosive sports require anaerobic power and strength and attract athletes of mesomorphic or endomorphic morphology. However, in reality, most sports require a range of qualities and are suited to a range of individuals of very different athletic capacities.

3.2 A Definition of Sport

What exactly do we understand by 'sport'? This popular activity may be defined as 'all forms of physical and sporting activity, which, whether through organised participation or not, aims to improve physical and psychological condition; to develop social relationships and to obtain competition results regardless of sporting level' (Comité Des Ministres 1992). Sport is therefore not limited to high-level participation. It is enjoyed by all.

Indeed, the global impact of sport on society is portrayed in the law. For example, in France, the National Code of Sport insists upon the importance of participation beyond the physical component. It emphasises its role in education and cultural and social integration (Code du Sport 2017). *SportAccord*, the largest association of international sporting federations, defines sport by the following elements:

S.C. Budd, J.-C. Egea, *Sport and Oral Health*, DOI 10.1007/978-3-319-53423-7_3

Table 3.1 The different categories of modern sport

Category of sport	Common examples
Physical	Athletics, rugby, handball, football, gymnastics, swimming
Motorised	Formula 1, motorcycling
Coordination	Archery, rifle shooting
Animal supported	Equestrian, polo
Mind	Chess

Sport:

1. Should include an element of competition
2. Should not rely on any element of 'luck' specifically integrated into the sport
3. Should not be judged to pose an undue risk to the health and safety of its athletes or participants
4. Should in no way be harmful to any living creature
5. Should not rely on equipment that is provided by a single supplier

A realm of activities is encompassed under the title of sport. The most precise classification of different sports is also given by SportAccord (2015). Sports are categorised as being physical, motorised, of coordination, animal supported and of the mind (Table 3.1). Sports may be also a combination of these criteria. As mentioned, sport implies an element of competition, either between teams or individuals.

3.3 A Clarification of Physical Activity, Sport and Exercise

Sport, exercise and physical activity are closely linked. However, strictly speaking, they are different. *Physical activity* may be defined as any *voluntary* action that exerts the body harder than at rest. Examples range from doing housework to dancing. *Exercise* is a form of physical activity, but is *specifically planned, structured and repetitive*. Examples include recreational jogging and swimming. *Sport* involves both physical activity and exercise. Here, the main difference is the *instigation of rules* that govern play, specific training programmes to improve performance and a degree of competition.

3.4 The Connection Between Different Types of *Physical* Sports

Physical sports cover a wide spectrum of activities, from the explosive to endurance. Endurance sports require a moderate effort over a prolonged period of time, whereas explosive sports entail short bursts of high intensity. Physiologically speaking, long-distance running and weightlifting, for example, have little in common. However, in reality, this distinction is not as clear-cut. The long-distance runner will require an explosive burst at the end of a race, and the weightlifter will require endurance to lift increasingly heavy weights during competition.

Many popular team games and racquet sports require both an endurance base and intensive bursts. The perfect example is that of a footballer. At elite level, the

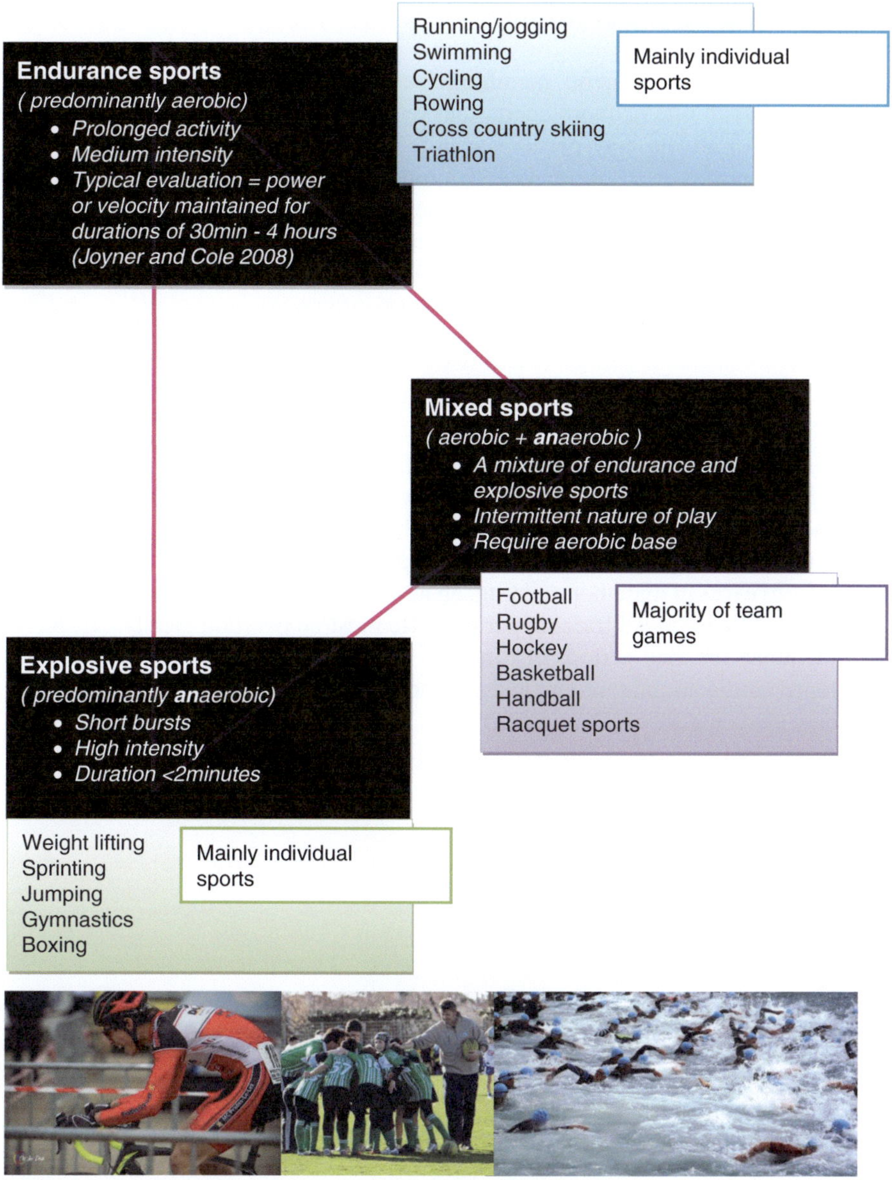

Fig. 3.1 The physiological interrelationship between popular sports

average footballer covers 10 km in a 90-min game. This is a mixture of steady aerobic exercise superimposed with explosive anaerobic bursts, which include kicking, jumping, sprinting and tackling (Stolen et al. 2005). Different sports therefore require a mixture of physiological qualities, which is reflected in their training principles to reach peak performance.

Figure 3.1 provides a simple classification of popular modern-day physical sports by their physical requirements.

3.5 Athletes: A Definition

Derived from Greek ἀθλητὴς, an athlete is a general term given to an individual who *competes* in one or more sports that require physical strength, speed and/or endurance. An athlete may participate in team or individual sports, as a professional, semi-professional or amateur. Training programmes differ in intensity and frequency of sessions, according to the athlete's individual goals.

An athlete is therefore an individual of varying abilities, who regularly trains and participates competitively in a given sport. An athlete may be a recreational participant of organised events or an elite international competitor.

3.5.1 Which Sport for Which Athlete?

Sport is for everyone. To maximise the benefits for our physical and psychological wellbeing, regular exercise of any kind may well suffice. However, several elements influence the choice of sport if the aim is to become a top-level athlete. These factors may be considered as environmental, psychological and physiological. For example, to excel in marathon running, an athlete ideally needs access to a running club to meet like-minded training partners. He must be psychologically capable of training alone for long periods of time and would physically benefit from a well-developed cardiovascular system and ectomorphic morphology.

These elements are neatly summarised in Fig. 3.2, which shows the main prerequisites required to excel in different types of sport.

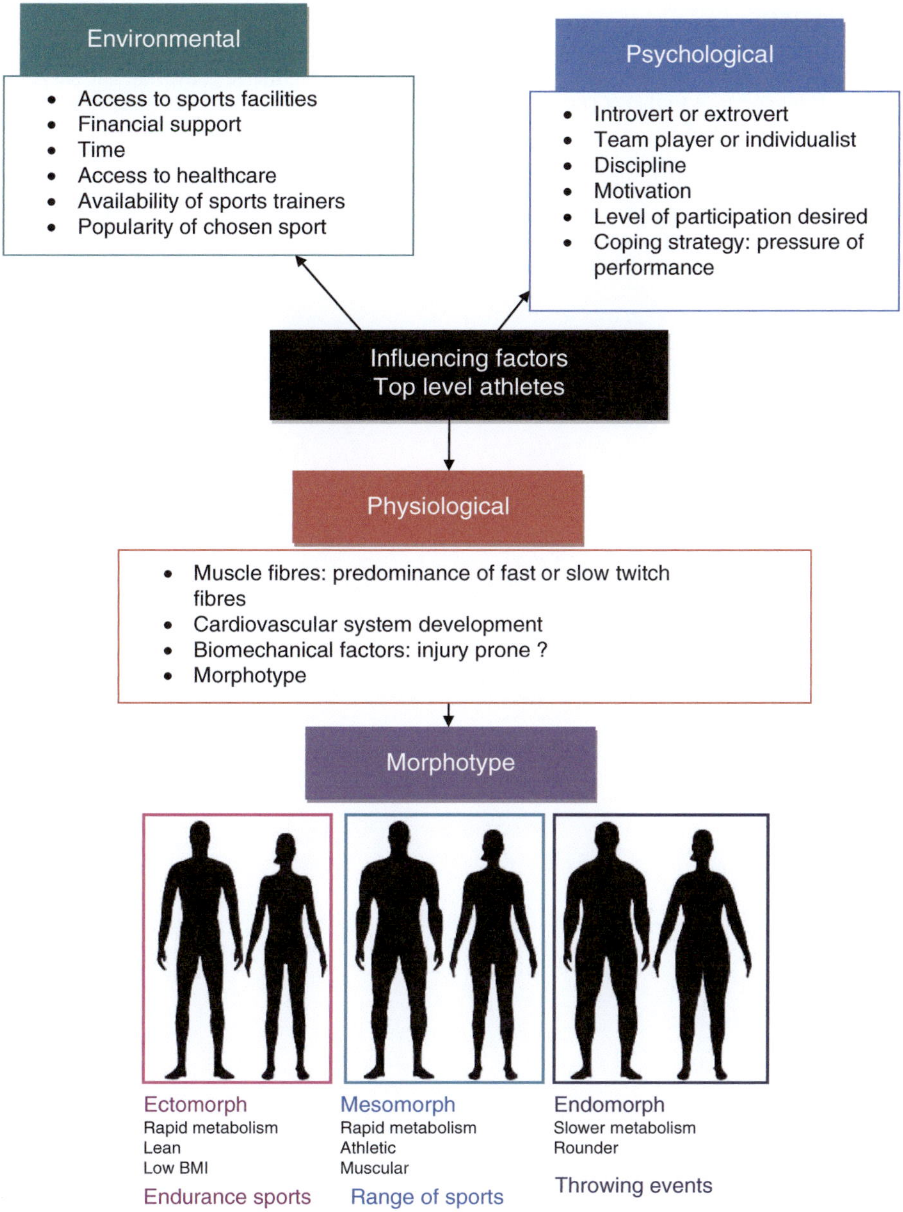

Fig. 3.2 Influential factors in becoming a top-level athlete

References

Code du Sport (2017) Vol. Article L. pp 100–101. https://www.legifrance.gouv.fr/affichCodeArticle.do?cidTexte=LEGITEXT000006071318&idArticle=LEGIARTI000006547489(2006). Accessed Nov 2015

Comité Des Ministres aux Etats Membres sur la Charte Européenne du Sport Revisée (1992) Recommandation 13 rév. http://www.coe.int/t/dg4/epas/source/11666. Accessed 20 Dec 2015

SportAccord: definition of Sport (2015) http://www.sportaccord.com/about/membership/definition-of-sport.php. Accessed 24 Jan 2016

Stølen T, Karim C, Carlo C, Ulrik W (2005) Physiology of soccer: an update. Sports Med (Auckl, NZ) 36(6):501–536

Understanding Training for Physical Sports and Its Physiological Demands

4

4.1 Introduction

In order to understand why athletes may be more susceptible to compromised oral health, it is essential to have an understanding of the physiological principles of training. Such knowledge gives an insight into the extra stresses placed upon an athlete's body and explains why the athlete modifies his behaviour to further improve performance.

Four key elements of training can be applied to the majority of sports. These consist of aerobic capacity development, amelioration of exercise economy, increasing an individual's lactate threshold and enhancement of their anaerobic capacity.

However, athletes are also faced with obstacles that can limit their performance. These can be immediate, linked to training and to competition, such as the depletion of muscle glycogen stores. Equally, limiting factors can arise over longer time periods and include fatigue, illness, malnutrition and stress. An athlete needs to overcome these hurdles. Coping strategies may well enable the athlete to reach optimal fitness and performance, but potential risks to oral health are involved.

4.2 The Aim of Training

Regardless of level of participation or ability, the aim of training is to improve an individual's performance in their chosen sport. It must therefore be sport specific and of a progressive nature and incorporate adequate rest or cross training to avoid injury and burnout.

The choice of sport determines the specific training goals. If we take the example of a 10 km runner, the aims are to:

(a) Increase his velocity at maximal oxygen uptake (vVO2 max), therefore improving his maximum aerobic speed.
(b) Increase the duration he can run at this speed (endurance).

S.C. Budd, J.-C. Egea, *Sport and Oral Health*, DOI 10.1007/978-3-319-53423-7_4

These two principles can be simply illustrated by an athlete who runs 10 km in 40 min (Fig. 4.1).

If we take a second example, that of a footballer during a match, certain similarities exist with the 10 km runner (Fig. 4.2). Physically, he too needs to maximise his aerobic velocity and increase his endurance to maintain it over the duration of the match. However, the graphics change due to the more explosive nature of his efforts and the intermittent nature of play. The footballer must develop his anaerobic velocity (without oxygen) in order to tackle or chase the ball. These bursts are more frequent than in the case of the 10 km runner, so speed endurance in anaerobic conditions is also an important focus.

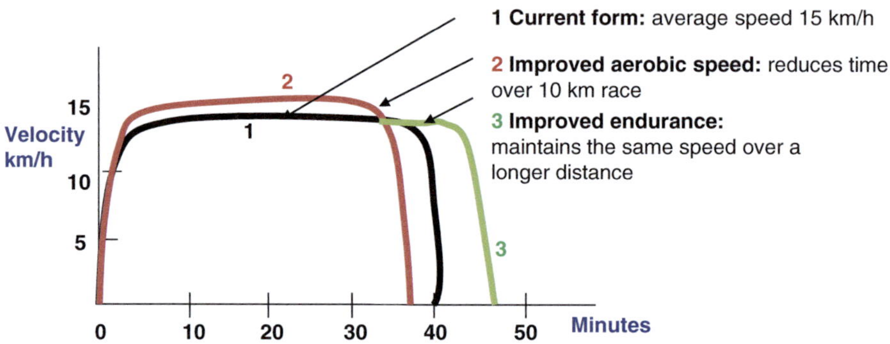

Fig. 4.1 A schematic illustration of the aim of 10 km running

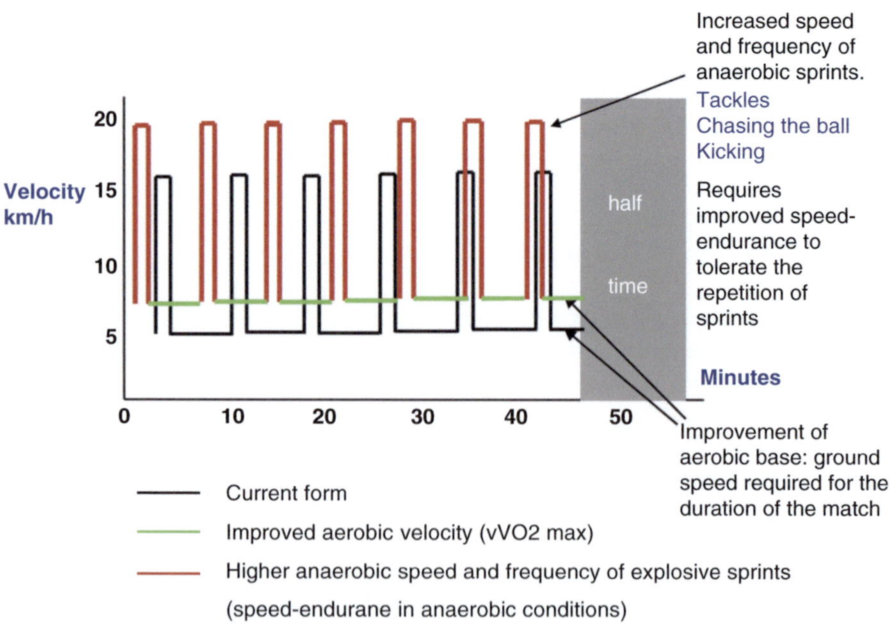

Fig. 4.2 The training aims for a footballer

4.3 The Four Key Parameters of Physical Training

In order to improve performance in *any* sport, the training schedule of an athlete must therefore address 4 key parameters of fitness (Jones and Carter 2000):

(i) Aerobic capacity (VO2max)
(ii) Exercise economy
(iii) Lactate/ventilatory threshold
(iv) Maximal anaerobic velocity

To summarise the general principles of training, Fig. 4.3 associates the components which form the basis of an effective plan.

The progress of an endurance athlete who solely focuses on his aerobic capacity will stagnate compared to the endurance athlete who incorporates a varied programme. Improved muscle force, biomechanics and anaerobic capacity ensure an efficient, finely tuned neuromuscular system which can consequently train at ease in aerobic conditions.

Inversely, the sprinter who improves the oxygenation and function of his cardiovascular system is better equipped to deal with decreased oxygen availability during his intense efforts and minimises accumulation of waste products such as lactic acid.

Another element of fitness often overlooked is flexibility. Increased flexibility helps posture, reduces muscular and articular tension, reduces injury risk and ultimately improves performance (Joyner and Coyle 2008; Rabadan et al. 2011).

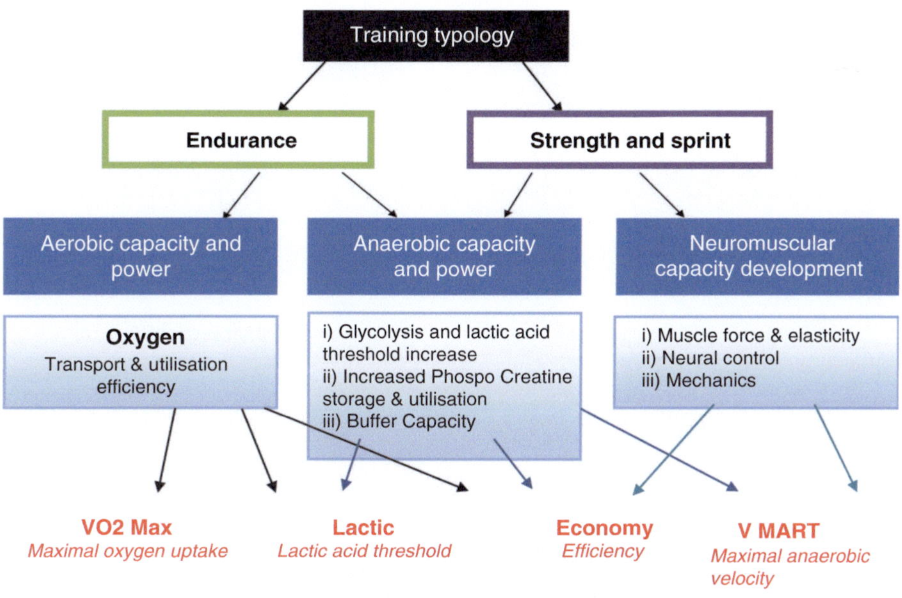

Fig. 4.3 Physiological components of training and performance

4.4 Limitations of Athletic Performance

4.4.1 During Competition and Training

A major obstacle in training, whether for an explosive or endurance sport, is the production of lactic acid. The lactic acid threshold is reached in response to insufficient oxygen reserves during intensive sustained muscular effort. Consequently, there is an exponential accumulation of hydrogen ions (H+) in the bloodstream. The athlete's power and velocity dramatically drops and the sensation of having 'nothing left' installs. A second problem is that of hyperthermia, via dehydration and endogenic heat increase in response to maximal physical exertion (under control of the central nervous system, *CNS*). The final obstacle to performance, during particularly long training sessions, is the depletion of glycogen stores commonly referred to as 'hitting the wall' – this mainly applies to sustained exercise lasting 30 minutes or more (Coyle 1999; Jeukendrup 2011).

4.4.2 Long-Term Limitations

Multifactorial, the main causes are linked to the disrespect of the progressive nature of training. They include inadequate nutrition and 'too much too soon with insufficient recovery '. Equally inhibiting are injury, illness, accidents, stress and the time balance of family and work (Coyle 1999; Jeukendrup 2011). Figure 4.4 summarises the limitations of sporting performance. Both the immediate and long-term elements are recapitulated.

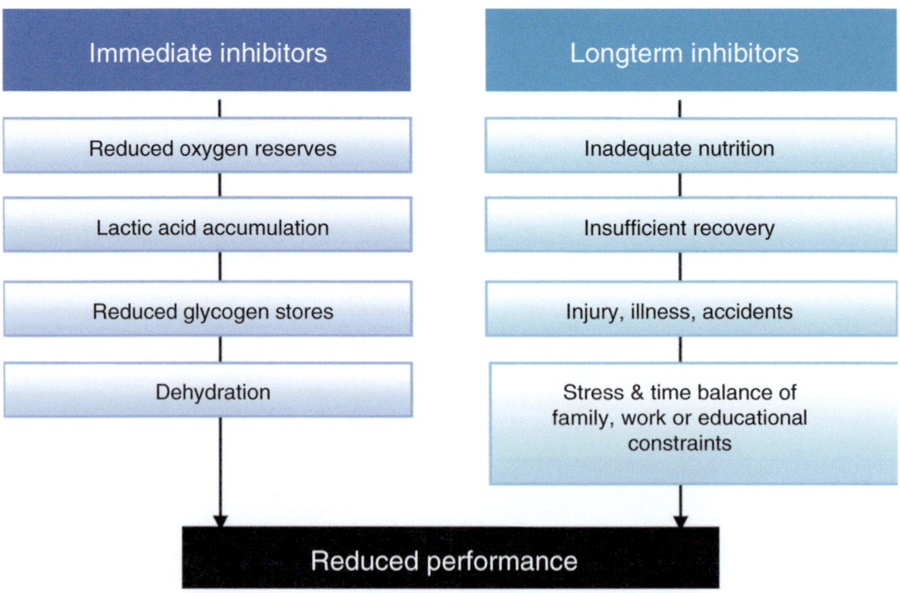

Fig. 4.4 The limitations of training and performance

References

Coyle EF (1999) Physiological determinants of endurance exercise performance. J Sci Med Sport 2(3):181–189

Jeukendrup AE (2011) Nutrition for endurance sports: marathon, triathlon, and road cycling. J Sports Sci 29(Suppl 1):91–99

Jones AM, Carter H (2000) The effect of endurance training on parameters of aerobic fitness. Sports Med (Auckl, NZ) 29:373–386

Joyner MJ, Coyle EF (2008) Endurance exercise performance: the physiology of champions. J Physiol 586(1):35–44

Rabadán M, Díaz V, Calderón FJ, Benito PJ, Peinado AB, Maffulli N (2011) Physiological determinants of speciality of elite middle- and long-distance runners. J Sports Sci 29(9):975–982

Part II

Oral Health and Sports-Related Risks

A variety of sports-related risk factors are poised to threaten the oral health of athletes. It is therefore fundamental to identify them and increase awareness of both the sporting population and health professionals alike.

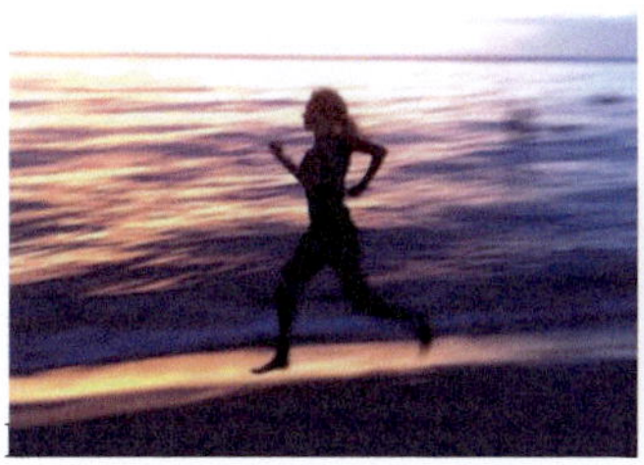
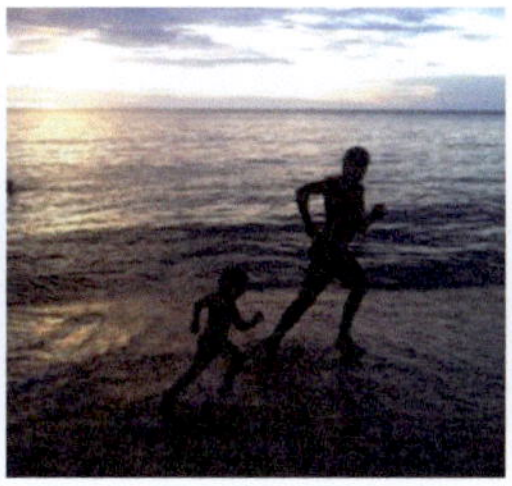
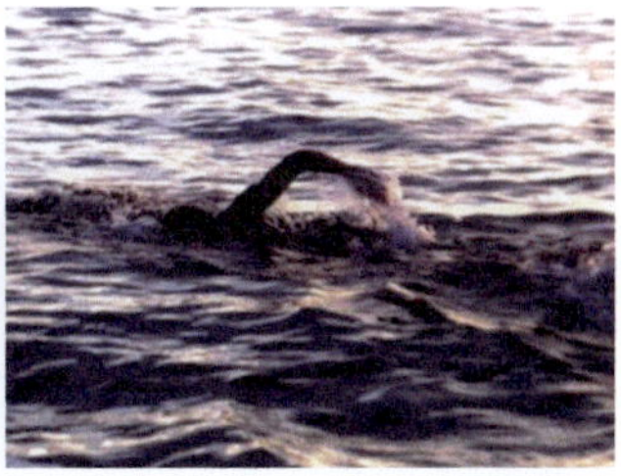

The Importance of Oral Health and Athletes

5

5.1 Introduction

Oral health is a vital component of our physiological and psychological wellbeing. However, current statistics reveal an alarming prevalence of oral diseases on a global scale, the majority of which are preventable if intercepted at an early stage.

In response, the World Health Organisation has issued pertinent guidelines which aim to improve the oral health of a range of populations. These include the improvement of dental care infrastructures and education in personal oral hygiene.

Known for high levels of fitness, athletes are not immune to oral health problems. Indeed, they represent a population particularly vulnerable to certain oral health lesions, which have been exacerbated by sports-related oral health risk factors. These risks include hyposalivation (hyposialia) and prejudicial eating habits during sporting effort, dental traumatology, training at high intensity, self-medication and the lack of prioritisation of oral healthcare. Identification of these oral health risks is an essential component in the management of active patients.

5.2 Oral Health

Oral health is essential to general health, quality of life and general wellbeing. It is defined by the World Health Organization as: ' A state of being free from mouth and facial pain, oral and throat cancer, oral infection and sores, periodontal (gum) disease, tooth decay, tooth loss, and other diseases and disorders that limit an individual's capacity in biting, chewing, smiling, speaking, and psychosocial wellbeing'.

'The most common oral diseases which affect people in both developed and less developed countries are dental cavities, periodontal (gum) disease, oral cancer, oral infectious diseases, trauma from injuries, and hereditary lesions' (WHO 2012). Worldwide, about 30% of people aged 65 to 74 are without natural teeth. Severe periodontal diseases affect up to 20% of adults aged 35 to 44 and almost 100% of adults have dental caries.

S.C. Budd, J.-C. Egea, *Sport and Oral Health*, DOI 10.1007/978-3-319-53423-7_5

5.3 Risk Factors and Oral Health: On a Global Scale

The main risk factors that aggravate oral diseases are also responsible for exacerbating the world's four leading noncommunicable chronic diseases – cancer, diabetes, cardiovascular illnesses and chronic respiratory syndromes. These risk factors are smoking, an unbalanced diet and harmful alcohol abuse. For oral diseases, poor oral hygiene is an additional hazard. These factors are governed by the environmental and social context. Unfortunately, oral disease is significantly higher amongst disadvantaged populations where access to dental treatment is limited (WHO 2016).

5.4 Reducing Oral Health Risks: Guidelines from the WHO

To achieve improved oral health, the WHO emphasises the importance of developing global policies in oral health promotion, which highlights the role of prevention. In fact, oral health should form part of an overall strategy for health promotion and chronic disease prevention. Table 5.1 illustrates the measures to be employed in order to combat the prevalence of oral disease (WHO 2012).

Table 5.1 Guidelines from the WHO to improve oral health on a global scale

Risk factor	Measure to improve oral health
Unbalanced diet and nutritional deficiencies	Decrease sugar intake Reduction of fizzy drinks Increased consumption of fruit and vegetables to help protect against oral cancer
Tobacco and alcohol abuse	Reduction of both helps reduce the risk of oral cancers, periodontal disease and tooth loss
Oral hygiene	Fluoride toothpaste Mouthwashes
Environment	Safe physical environments
Sports and motor vehicle equipment	Usage of protective equipment in sports to prevent orofacial injury
Dental care infrastructure	Schemes to target especially the older generation living in isolated rural areas
Oral health policies	Control of risks to oral health Focus on community-based projects for disadvantaged populations
Fluoride	Encourage National Health Authorities: fluoride programmes Schemes for water fluoridation Fluoride toothpastes Aliments containing fluoride – salt/milk Topical application fluoride

Source: Based on guidelines of the World Health Organisation (2012)

5.5 The Specific Case of Athletes and Oral Health

Athletes are evidently subjected to the same oral health risk factors as the general population. Ironically, with focus on exceptional physical fitness, the oral health of many athletes is often sidelined. It is as if the buccal cavity is a separate entity on the human body – only when in pain does its importance become paramount.

Athletes are also predisposed to certain oral health risk factors directly linked to their participation in sport. These risks are linked to the demands of exercise and training on the human body. Multifaceted, they include sugar loading during training and competition, high-volume and high-intensity training inducing immunological perturbations, lack of education and prioritisation of oral health, insufficient access to dental care, medication and even the psychological makeup of the individual athlete.

A study on New Zealand elite triathletes highlights certain sports-related oral health risks. These high-level athletes were evaluated as high-risk candidates for both dental erosion and dental caries due to their high consumption of sugar-rich food and acidic drinks during training. A total of 84% consumed sports drinks, and 94% ate during sessions. Interestingly, *only 3%* were *conscious* of their detrimental behaviour towards oral health – indicating a lack of knowledge or education in oral health issues despite an accentuated awareness of general health (Bryant et al. 2011).

It is important to appreciate that these risk factors are not limited to oral hard and soft tissues. Training and performance can also be adversely affected. The propagation of oral infection, bad posture arising from dental malocclusion and dental pain are all linked to diminished sporting capacity. In addition, compromised oral health can have repercussions on an athlete's confidence and their quality of life. Figure 5.1 provides a simple overview of these risks; eight major themes are identified.

5.6 Regulatory Medical Surveillance of Sport: A European Example

Athletes of all levels are subjected to certain medical controls if they wish to participate in sporting events. Even recreational participants who rarely compete are strongly advised to be controlled by their general practitioner.

The individual athlete, non-affiliated to a club, must often produce a medical certificate to participate in an organised sporting event, in the prevention of public health accidents. However, given the nonvital implications of dental disease, dental check-ups are not imposed at this level.

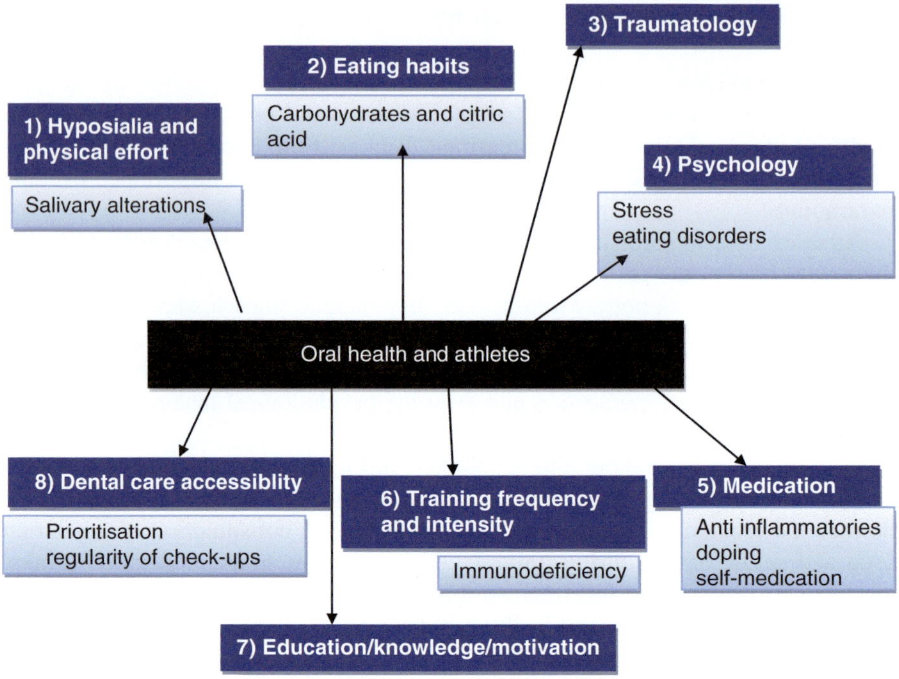

Fig. 5.1 A summary of the oral health risk factors affecting athletes

5.7 The Role of Sports Federations: The French Example

In 2012, 16 million people, approximately one quarter of the entire French population, were affiliated to chartered sporting federations (Ministère de Droits 2014). How exactly are these sports federations involved in the medical surveillance of their athletes? They intervene at three levels:

1. They inform and prevent doping amongst athletes, in collaboration with the national anti-doping body, here the 'Association Francaise de Lutte contre le Dopage (AFLD)'.
2. To be affiliated, the individual must produce a valid medical certificate of eligibility to participate in the given sport.
3. For elite sportsmen and women: as from their initial registration, obligatory medical exams are frequently required. These include an annual *dental check-up* to assure oral health (*Code du Sport Art L231–5, 6, 7; . R231–4, 7)* (Depiesse 2010).

This check-up focuses on the athlete's medical and sporting history. It details prevention and a clinical examination of hygiene, the presence of infections, hard and soft tissue examinations and the investigation of oral functions and parafunctions.

References

Bryant S, McLaughlin K, Morgaine K, Drummond B (2011) Elite athletes and oral health. Int J Sports Med 32:720–724

Depiesse F (2010) Table ronde 1: Suivi réglementaire et sanitaire au sein des féderations. Conférence Nationale Médicale Interfédérale du CNOSF. http://franceolympique.com/files/File/actions/sante/colloques/suivireglementaireetsanitaire.pdf. Accessed Feb 2015

Ministère de Droits Des Femmes, De la Ville, De la Jeunesse et Des Sports. Les chiffres clés du sport (2014) http://www.sports.gouv.fr/IMG/pdf/ccs_juin_2014.pdf. Accessed Oct 2015

World Health Organisation (2012) Oral health fact sheet number 318. http://www.who.int/mediacentre/factsheets/fs318/en/. Accessed 15 July 2016

World Health Organisation (2016) Strategies and approaches in oral disease prevention and health promotion. http://www.who.int/oral_health/strategies/cont/en/. Accessed 16 July 2016

6 Oral Health Risk Factor: Nutrition of Athletes

6.1 Introduction

The first major risk to oral health is an athlete's diet. This is somewhat surprising, given the attention placed upon nutrition for peak performance. In order to understand potential oral health consequences linked to athletes' eating habits, we must be aware of their energy demands, both quantitatively and qualitatively, to improve performance. Athletes have much higher energy requirements than the general population and also require a higher proportion of certain nutrients potentially hazardous to oral health if consumed to excess. Indeed, popular sports supplements are often rich in carbohydrates and acidic fruit extracts. The frequent ingestion of these nutrients during physical exertion potentialises the risk of hard dental tissue lesions, notably dental caries and erosion development.

Equipped with knowledge of the nutritional demands of athletes, the dental practitioner is better placed to identify those at high risk, to educate, inform and implement prevention strategies adapted to their athletic patients (Joyner and Coyle 2008; Jeukendrup 2011).

6.2 Energy Pathways (Metabolism) of Physical Exertion

During physical exertion, the body converts chemical energy stored in nutrients into mechanical energy and waste products. However, the source of this chemical energy and its transformation into energy for movement varies according to the intensity and duration of the exercise.

Explosive sports require a rapidly available source of energy. This is provided by the anaerobic pathway (without oxygen). Muscle reserves of creatine phosphate supply energy for up to 10 s – the main source for 60 m sprinters or weightlifters, for example. Muscle glycogen and glucose then take the relay for intense efforts up to 3 min.

S.C. Budd, J.-C. Egea, *Sport and Oral Health*, DOI 10.1007/978-3-319-53423-7_6

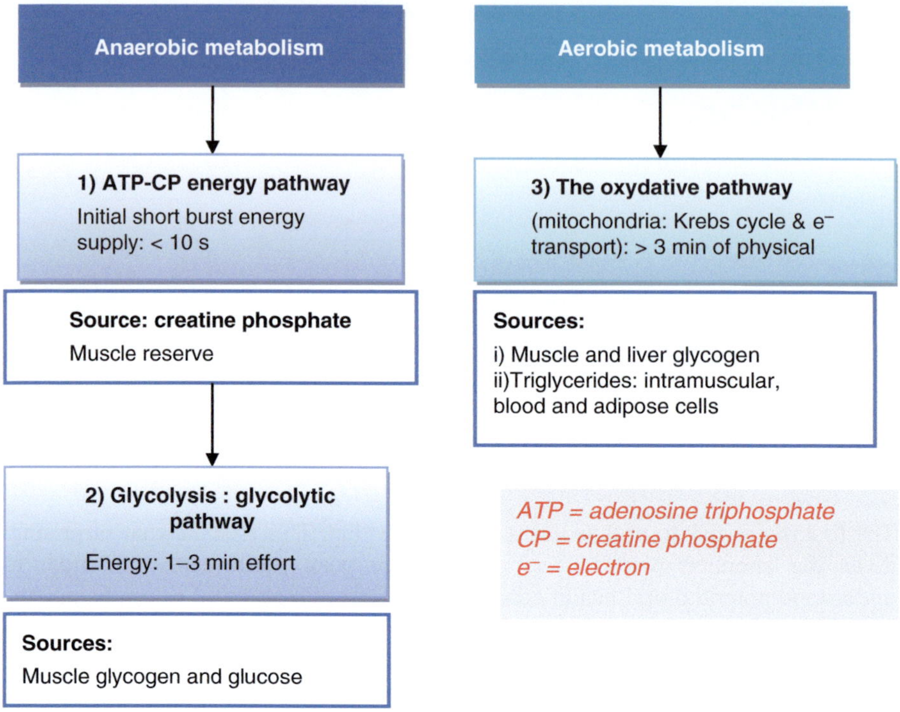

Fig. 6.1 Energy pathways of physical exertion in exercise and sport. *ATP* adenosine triphosphate, *CP* creatine phosphate, *e⁻* electron

Prolonged exercise relies on aerobic metabolism. Oxygen is required. A well-developed cardiovascular system acts as a motor to sustain physical exertion over a longer period of time.

Aerobic metabolism dominates endurance events, and anaerobic pathways the more explosive sports. However, in reality these complimentary energy pathways are closely interrelated. Figure 6.1 summarises these different energetic pathways.

6.3 The Energy Consumption of Athletes (Quantitative)

Considerably higher than sedentary individuals, the athlete consumes more energy more often. The athlete's energy requirement during intensive training may be up to ten times higher.

6.3.1 Quantitative Energy Expenditure of a Moderately Active Adult

The total daily energy expenditure (24 h) of a given human being is the sum of:

(a) *Basal metabolic rate (BMR)*: which assures all bodily functions (60–75%), approximately 1200 Kcal

(b) *Thermic effect of food*: post prandial augmentation of body temperature, dependent on the type of nutrient consumed (10%)
(c) *Non-activity thermogenesis*
(d) *Thermal effect of physical activity*: planned participation in sport and spontaneous physical activity such as shivering

An averagely active woman aged between 19 and 50 needs a daily calorific intake of approximately 2200Kcal, while an average man needs up to 2900 Kcal (American Dietetic Association 2000).

6.3.2 Energy Requirements of Athletes in Different Sports

The specific energy requirements of athletes (measured in KJ or Kcal) depend on numerous variables. These include intrinsic factors such as weight, sex, age and the intensity of exertion. Equally important are extrinsic environmental factors, including the weather conditions and terrain. Regardless of the sport, calorific needs increase dramatically during physical effort.

A compilation of energy expenditure values in hundreds of activities, ranging from sleeping to vigorous uphill cross-country skiing, was originally created by Ainsworth et al. (2000). It has since been revised to include 821 different activities. The unit given is known as the metabolic equivalent (MET) value score. *One MET = 1 Kcal/kg/h (4.184 KJ/kg/h)* (Ainsworth et al. 2000, 2011). Table 6.1 gives an insight into the energy requirements of different sports and activities (Ainsworth et al. 2000, 2011).

Let us take the example of a 70 kg male playing basketball for a total of 60 min. His average energy requirement is $8 \times 70 \times 1 = 560$ Kcal. Now if we take the same player, sitting down reading, he consumes less: $1.3 \times 70 \times 1 = 91$ Kcal. He requires approximately *six times* more energy for his game (Table 6.1).

In fact, in periods of intensive training, an athlete may require anywhere up to 10,000 Kcal/day. These huge energetic demands have several potential repercussions on oral health. An increased need for energy means more food and fluid more

Table 6.1 A comparison of energy expenditure in daily activities and sport (Ainsworth et al. 2000, 2011)

Activity	MET score (Kcal/kg/h)
Sleeping	0.9
Sedentary activities	1–1.5
Standing	2.3
Walking	3.5–5
Tennis	7
Basketball	8
Beach volleyball	8
Competitive football/soccer	9
Swimming	7–11
Rugby	10
Running 10 min/mile	10
Running 6 min/mile	16
Cross-country skiing	14–16.5

often. Often loaded with carbohydrates and even acidic nutrients, we begin to unravel the core of this oral health risk. Athletes have a higher individualised risk of caries (IRC) and vulnerability to dental erosions – due to the frequent consumption of sports compliments *during* sporting activity.

6.4 Specific Nutrition of Athletes

An athlete therefore needs to alter his dietary intake to meet the increased demands of training and competition to maximise both performance and recovery. The energy, nutrient and fluid recommendations for active adults and competitive athletes are listed in Fig. 6.2 which is based on national dietetic guidelines (American Dietetic Association 2000; Peinado et al. 2013). An athlete obviously needs to

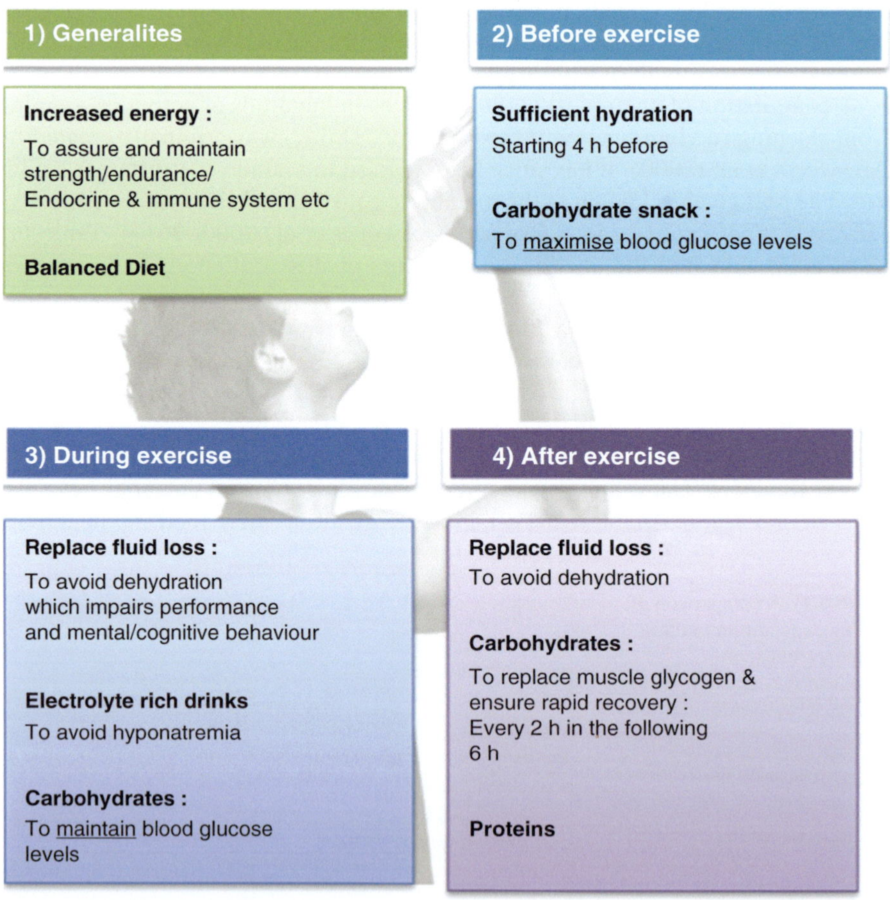

Fig. 6.2 Specifics of nutrition for athletes during physical exercise

follow a balanced diet, but must pay attention to his hydration, energy levels and sources of energy during exercise. Adapted to physical performance, it is not necessarily appropriate for optimal oral health.

A prime example is that of an endurance athlete. Let us take the example of a cyclist going for a 50 km ride. According to these recommendations, he should ideally start regularly ingesting carbohydrate-rich foods and drinks 4 h prior to effort, during the event and even up to 6 h later to replenish his sources (American Dietetic Association 2000).

6.5 The Risk to Oral Health: Dental Caries and Erosion

6.5.1 Sports Supplements

Highly commercialised sports drinks, energy bars and gels are becoming increasingly popular during both training and competition. The drinks contain relatively high amounts of carbohydrates (sugars), salt and citric acid (fruit), whereas the food supplements are loaded mainly with carbohydrates (Noble et al. 2011). All supplements aim to improve performance. However, frequent consumption of these dietary products places the athlete at a higher risk of dental erosions and exercise-dependent dental caries.

6.5.2 The Risk of Dental Caries: The Need for a 'Sugar Fix'

It is the high sugar (carbohydrate) content of most sports supplements which increases the risk of this infectious disease. Bacterial fermentation of these sugars produces an acidic byproduct, which causes demineralisation of enamel when the pH of the dental surface descends below 5.5. In normal circumstances, this process is reversible and entails remineralisation of the affected surface. However, specific eating habits during sporting activity can increase the risk of a continuous carious process (World Sugar Research Organisation 2011).

6.5.2.1 Increasing the Risk: Frequent Ingestion of Carbohydrates

The aforementioned cycle of demineralisation-mineralisation is disrupted by *frequent snacking* of sports supplements, particularly in the absence of adequate oral hygiene. This reduces the buffering capacity and remineralisation potential of the oral environment. Not a new concept, Gustaffson (1954) showed that *frequency* of sugar consumption was far more important in influencing dental caries than the *amount*. Figure 6.3 illustrates exactly how often an athlete should ingest supplements to improve performance, with reference to a semi marathon run in 2 h (American Dietetic Association 2000).

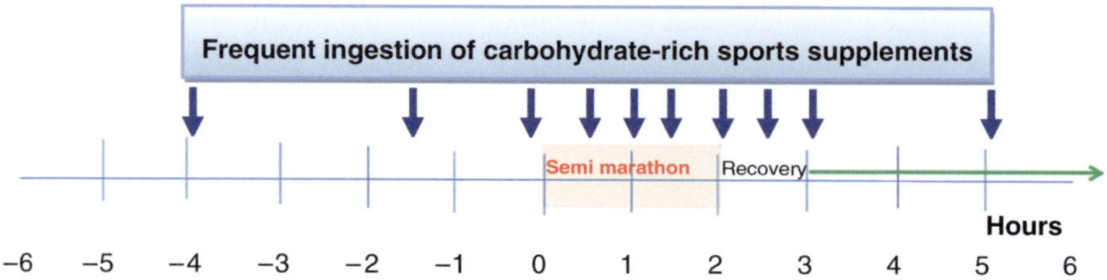

Fig. 6.3 High-frequency ingestion of carbohydrates during an endurance event

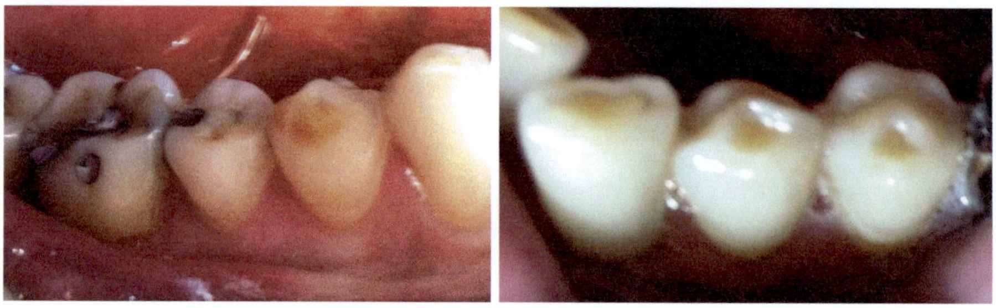

Fig. 6.4 Examples of dental erosion

6.5.3 The Erosive Potential of Sports Drinks

Due to their high fruit, hence citric acid, content, sports drinks facilitate enamel and dentin erosion. An athlete typically drinks small sips every 30 minutes during a given sporting event, as this equates to the diminution of his muscle glycogen reserves. Unfortunately, the buffering of oral acidity becomes an elusive concept during prolonged aerobic exercise. Demineralisation is constantly reactivated (Perez 2006) and the process of dental erosion accelerated (Fig. 6.4).

6.5.4 Summary: Athletes Particularly at Risk from Dental Caries or Erosion

It may be concluded that athletes are therefore particularly at risk from dental caries or erosion if they:

1. Frequently consume (snacking) sports supplements, essentially made of rapid sugars
2. Frequently drink sports drinks of a high carbohydrate and fruit content (citric acid)
3. Participate in several prolonged efforts, resulting in frequent episodes of hyposalivation and impairment of saliva's protection against enamel demineralisation
4. Are subject of common causal factors of the general population: bad oral hygiene/dental morphology/education/attitude

References

Ainsworth BE, Haskell WL, Whitt MC, Irwin ML, Swartz AM, Strath SJ, O'Brien WL et al (2000) Compendium of physical activities: an update of activity codes and MET intensities. Med Sci Sports Exerc 32:498–504

Ainsworth BE, Haskell WL, Herrmann SD, Meckes N, Bassett DR, Tudor-Locke C, Greer JL, Vezina J, Whitt-Glover MC, Leon AS (2011) Compendium of physical activities: a second update of codes and MET values. Med Sci Sports Exerc 43:1575–1581

Gustaffson BE (1954) The Vipeholm dental caries study: survey of the literature on carbohydrates and dental caries. Acta Odontol Scand 11:207–231

Jeukendrup AE (2011) Nutrition for endurance sports: marathon, triathlon, and road cycling. J Sports Sci 29(Suppl 1):91–99

Joyner MJ, Coyle EF (2008) Endurance exercise performance: the physiology of champions. J Physiol 586:35–44

Noble WH, Donovan TE, Geissberger M (2011) Sports drinks and dental erosion. J Calif Dent Assoc 39:233–238

Peinado A, Miguel B, Rojo-Tirado A, Benito P (2013) Sugar and exercise: its importance in athletes. Nutr Hosp 28(Suppl 4):48–56

Perez S (2006) Dents et pratiques alimentaires chez les sportifs: Table Ronde odonto-stomatologie et sport. *Troisieme conference Nationale Médicale Interfédérale*. http://franceolympique.com/files/File/actions/sante/documentation/2007/3emeconf-2emetableronde.pdf. Accessed Nov 2015

Position of the American Dietetic Association (2000) Dieticians of Canada, and the American College of Sports Medicine: nutrition and athletic performance. J Am Diet Assoc 100(12):1543–1556

World Sugar Research Organisation (WSRO) (2011) Sugar and Dental Caries. http://www.wsro.org/AboutSugar/Sugardentalcaries.aspx. Accessed 15 July 2016

Oral Health Risk Factor: Cumulative Training and High-Intensity Sessions

7

7.1 Introduction

Can regular exercise and sport ever become too much of a 'good thing'? With regard to oral health, the two main considerations are cumulative weekly training time and the intensity at which the athlete trains. Studies have revealed a higher prevalence of certain dental lesions amongst athletes who train frequently. Evidently, a positive relationship exists between the time devoted to training and the exposure to oral health risks.

Equally important is the intensity at which an athlete exercises. If an athlete does not respect the progressive nature of his training schedules, adapted to his capacity, he is susceptible to fatigue, illness and eventual burnout.

The perfect illustration in the field of dentistry is the phenomenon of exercise-induced modulation of the immune system, due to unadapted, overzealous training. Classified as either acute or chronic perturbations, the athlete becomes susceptible to opportunistic infections, such as *Candida albicans* or herpes simplex. Equally, infections of the upper respiratory tract are common amongst endurance athletes. These are partly due to interference with immunoglobulin levels in saliva.

7.2 Cumulative Weekly Training

The greater the exposure to oral health risk factors, the greater the probability they become a reality. This may be considered as 'cumulative risk' and applies to all risk factors, whether psychological or physiological.

For example, a study by Frese et al. (2014) revealed a positive correlation between cumulative weekly training and caries prevalence. An increased frequency of carbohydrate consumption, associated to decreased saliva, was to blame. His findings are illustrated on the scatterplot of Spearman (Fig. 7.1).

S.C. Budd, J.-C. Egea, *Sport and Oral Health*, DOI 10.1007/978-3-319-53423-7_7

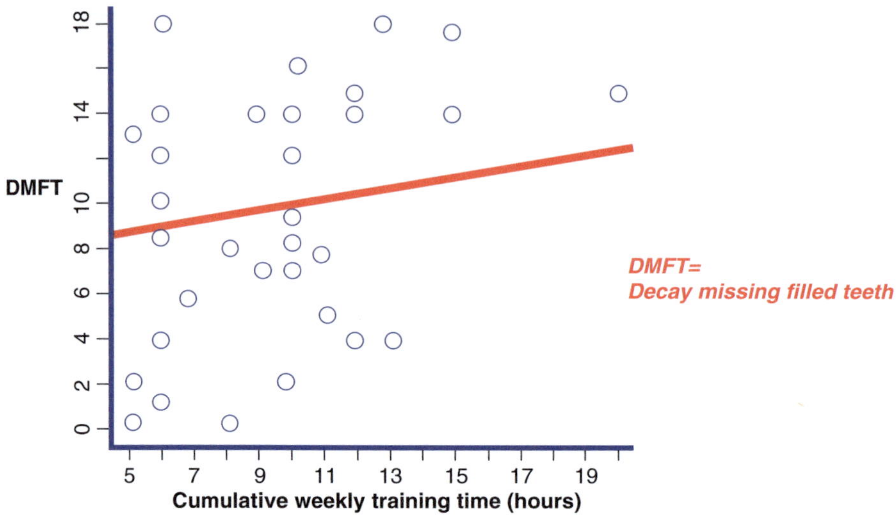

Fig. 7.1 The correlation between cumulative weekly training and tooth decay. *DMFT* decay missing filled teeth

7.3 Intensity of Training Coupled to Cumulation of Training

An increase in training intensity further exacerbates the risks to oral health. The terminology 'intensive training' implies that the body is not given sufficient recovery before the next session. Alternatively, more than 7 hours practice a week is classified as intensive. Such levels of participation are not limited to elite athletes. Endorphine release during physical exercise and noticeable corporal improvements can entice even the most recreational of participants to become addicted to sport. Some individuals can even become overly dependant on physical activity and exercise to an excessive degree. This abuse of exercise can be detrimental to both physical and psychological health (Raglin 1990).

A good example of adverse effects of intense training on the human body is the modulation of the immune system. Any deficiency of immunity renders the individual less capable to fight infection of the oral cavity or elsewhere.

7.3.1 Exercise-Induced Modulation of the Immune System: Risk Factor

Immune function is the result of a complex interaction of factors. These include physical, psychological and environmental elements (Gleeson 2006). With regard to sport, moderate exercise helps build immunity. It helps reduce chronic inflammation and is beneficial to people of all ages (Derek et al. 2008). Unfortunately, intensive exercise may be detrimental on a short and long-term basis. We distinguish two ways in which the immune system can be affected – temporarily or chronically.

7.3.1.1 Acute Versus Cumulative Immune System Modulation

A transient suppression of certain immunity parameters can result within the 72 hours following strenuous exercise. This becomes more acute if the athlete has a low fitness level, is badly trained (Frank et al. 2004), stressed and inadequately nutritioned for his sporting needs. The athlete becomes more vulnerable to acute and viral infections, as well as aging and cancer (Shephard and Shek 1994). Kakanis et al. (2010) revealed a short-term decrease in immune function followed intensive training in elite cyclists. They recorded a drop of lymphocyte numbers 2 hours post exercise, a mobilisation of neutrophils and an increased inflammatory response of cytokines. These findings supported their 'open window theory' of pathogen opportunity following strenuous exercise.

More menacing is a chronic accumulation of immunity deficiency over time. Prolonged periods of intensive training coupled to inadequate recovery result in subtle changes of several constituents of the immune system. These include modification of neutrophil function, serum, immunoglobulin and plasma glutamine concentration and even natural killer cytotoxic activity. The mucosal immune system response, responsible for upper respiratory tract infections, is commonly affected. Endurance athletes are particularly vulnerable due to their high-volume training schedules (Mackinnon 2000).

7.3.2 Sports-Related Immunomodulation and Dentistry

As for any other immunocompromised patient, a fatigued athlete is more vulnerable to opportunistic infections of the oral cavity. Such infections may be fungal, bacterial or viral in nature. Common culprits are *Candida albicans* and the herpes simplex (Fig. 7.2). According to Van Dyke and Hoop (1990), even a light impairment to neutrophil function increases the susceptibility of the vulnerable periodontium to infection.

The main antibody found in saliva, IgA, has been investigated by several scientists. It helps protect the oral cavity by inhibiting the adherence of microorganisms to both teeth and the oral epithelium. Any qualitative or quantitative interference with its presence therefore poses a risk of oral infection (Ryley et al. 1982). Indeed,

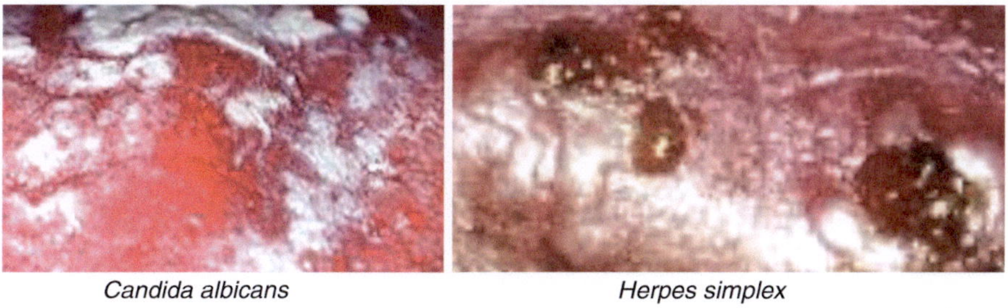

Fig. 7.2 Opportunistic infections of the oral cavity

numerous studies on competitive swimmers have reported a frequent lowering of their salivary immunoglobulin levels. These athletes are particularly vulnerable to infection when subjected to intense, repetitive training over several months (Gleeson 2006; Mackinnon and Hooper 1994).

References

Derek A, Sabljic TF, Baribeau BA, Haaland DA, Mukovozov IM, Hart LE (2008) Is regular exercise a friend or foe of the aging immune system? A systematic review. Clin J Sport Med Off J Can Acad Sport Med 18:539–548

Van Dyke TE, Hoop GA (1990) Neutrophil function and oral disease. Crit Rev Oral Biol Med Off Publ Am Assoc Oral Biol 1:2;117–133

Frank C, Mooren FC et al (2004) Exercise-induced apoptosis of lymphocytes depends on training status. Med Sci Sports Exerc 36:1476–1483

Frese CF, Frese S, Kuhlmann D, Saure D, Reljic HJ, Staehle HJ, Wolff D (2015) Effect of endurance training on dental erosion, caries, and saliva. Scand J Med Sci Sports 25(3):219–326

Gleeson M (2006) Immune system adaptation in elite athletes. Curr Opin Clin Nutr Metab Care 9: 659–665

Kakanis MW, Peake J, Brenu EW, Simmonds M, Gray B, Hooper SL, Marshall-Gradisnik SM (2010) The open window of susceptibility to infection after acute exercise in healthy young male elite athletes. Exerc Immunol Rev 16:119–137

Mackinnon LT (2000) Chronic exercise training effects on immune function. Med Sci Sports Exerc 32:369–376

Mackinnon LT, Hooper D (1994) Mucosal (Secretory) immune system responses to exercise of varying intensity and during overtraining. Int J Sports Med 15(Suppl 3):179–183

Raglin JS (1990) Exercise and mental health. Beneficial and detrimental effects. Sports Med (Auckl, NZ) 9:323–329

Ryley H, Vudhichamnong K, Walker DM (1982) The effect of secretory immunoglobulin A on the in-vitro adherence of the yeast *Candida albicans* to human oral epithelial cells. Arch Oral Biol 27:617–621

Shephard R, Shek P (1994) Potential impact of physical activity and sport on the immune system – a brief review. Br J Sports Med 28:247–255

Oral Health Risk Factor: Quantitative Salivary Alterations

8

8.1 Introduction

Both a qualitative and *quantitative* alteration of saliva's constituents have deleterious effects on the oral cavity. A decrease in saliva production during physical exertion, a phenomenon known as *hypo*salivation, or *xero*stomia in the case of complete interruption, is particularly detrimental.

Three processes are responsible for hyposalivation during sport. Firstly, stress associated to competition stimulates the sympathetic nervous system and reduces saliva secretion into the buccal cavity. Secondly, heat production and consequent transpiration during effort offset a negative feedback system to restore homeostasis. Saliva secretion is reduced. Thirdly, the exposition of the buccal cavity to external climatic elements induces evaporation at the surfaces of oral constituents.

Saliva is multifunctional. It is a lubricant and protects the oral cavity from infection and acid demineralisation. With regard to athletes, hyposalivation during physical effort exacerbates the risk of dental caries and erosion and opportunistic infections of the oral sphere.

8.2 Saliva Production During Physical Exertion

Hyposalivation during sporting activity is therefore a major risk to oral health (Fig. 8.1). This decrease in saliva not only interferes with oral functions, such as digestion and phonation, but predisposes the athlete to various oral infections. Furthermore, it aggravates demineralisation of hard dental surfaces. Acids remain stagnant in the oral cavity and the potential to remineralise affected dental surfaces becomes difficult. The athlete is therefore more vulnerable to both dental caries and dental erosion. In sport, hyposalivation is primarily due to three factors: stress (the anticipation of effort or competition), heat production during physical effort (thermogenesis), and buccal respiration. Consequently, the protective powers of

S.C. Budd, J.-C. Egea, *Sport and Oral Health*, DOI 10.1007/978-3-319-53423-7_8

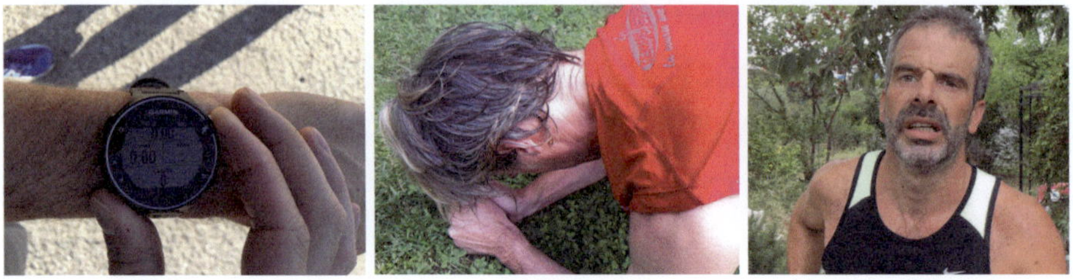

Fig. 8.1 Factors affecting saliva production

saliva are diminished or even lost. Fortunately, during physical exertion, this hyposalivation is of a temporary nature. However, problems arise when the frequency and intensity of training increases. Hyposalivation becomes a regular occurrence.

8.2.1 Stress: Stimulation of the Sympathetic Nervous System

The main culprit of hyposalivation during exercise is psychological, linked to the anxiety and stress of competition. In this context, it is the sympathetic nervous system, part of the autonomic nervous system, which regulates the secretion of saliva. It prepares the body for 'fright or flight', a physiological preparation to meet the demands of strenuous exercise. Consequently, during physical effort, cardiac and respiratory output increases, as does production of adrenaline, sweat and liver glucose. All functions deemed unessential are slowed, such as digestion and the production of saliva, hence the phenomenon of hyposalivation. Several studies have investigated the role of the sympathetic nervous system on saliva production in sport. Li and Gleeson (2004), for example, explored the relationship between cycling at a moderate intensity for 2 hour periods and saliva flux. It was concluded that sympathetic stimulation appeared to be strong enough to completely inhibit saliva flow rate of these athletes.

8.2.2 Heat Production and Homeostasis

A second reason for hyposalivation during physical effort is the elimination of body fluids to prevent internal overheating. Hydration levels of a given individual are an important influencing factor on salivary secretion. If the body's water content is reduced by 8%, saliva flow is virtually zero to conserve water (Dawes 1987).

So how does is participation in sport influence our hydration levels? Muscular contractions during exercise generate heat as a byproduct. This change in body temperature is then detected by the body's heat receptors, which inform the central nervous system (hypothalamus) of this alteration of homeostasis. In response, the hypothalamus stimulates a negative feedback system to restore body temperature. Vasodilation of blood vessels at the skin's surface permits evaporation of water and heat loss, as does fluid secretion by sweat glands. By time an athlete complains of thirst, substantial water loss has already occurred, to the point of interference with performance.

8.2.3 Buccal Respiration

A third factor in sport that influences hyposalivation is buccal respiration. Athletes adopt this particular form of respiration during prolonged physical exertion. Here, the salivary flux remains constant, but saliva is more readily evaporated from the surfaces of the buccal cavity (Lamendin 2004). This is due to exposure to external climatic elements. Figure 8.2 summarises the aetiology of hyposalivation during sporting effort.

8.3 Hyposalivation as a Risk for Oral Health: The Roles of Saliva

Water is the major constituent of saliva along with small but necessary levels of electrolytes. Other molecules with biological and biochemical properties essential to maintain the stomatognathic system physiology are also present. This is a complex mixture with many components, including proteins, glycoproteins and enzymes (Turner and Hiroshi 2002).

The diverse roles of saliva in the oral cavity are therefore due to its disposition and action. This chapter highlights the functions of saliva and how hyposalivation during physical exercise becomes an oral health risk for athletes.

Saliva facilitates taste, phonation and digestion, provides protection and humectation to oral mucosal structures and forms a protective organic pellicule on hard dental tissues (Gonsalez and Sung 2014). Over the years, saliva's roles have been discussed by numerous scientists, such as Mandel (1989), Levine (1993) and more recently Buzalaf et al. (2012). These complimentary studies have permitted a precise identification of salivary mechanisms which protect diverse elements of oral health. The protective roles of saliva in relation to *oral health* are summarised in Table 8.1.

8.3.1 Saliva, Oral Health and Sport

The phenomenon of hyposalivation during physical effort forms part of a symbiosis of hazards that can jeopardise the oral cavity (Levine 1993). The loss of saliva's protective properties increases the risk of dental erosion and caries from frequent supplement ingestion and the development of opportunistic infections linked to intensive training sessions (Fig. 8.3).

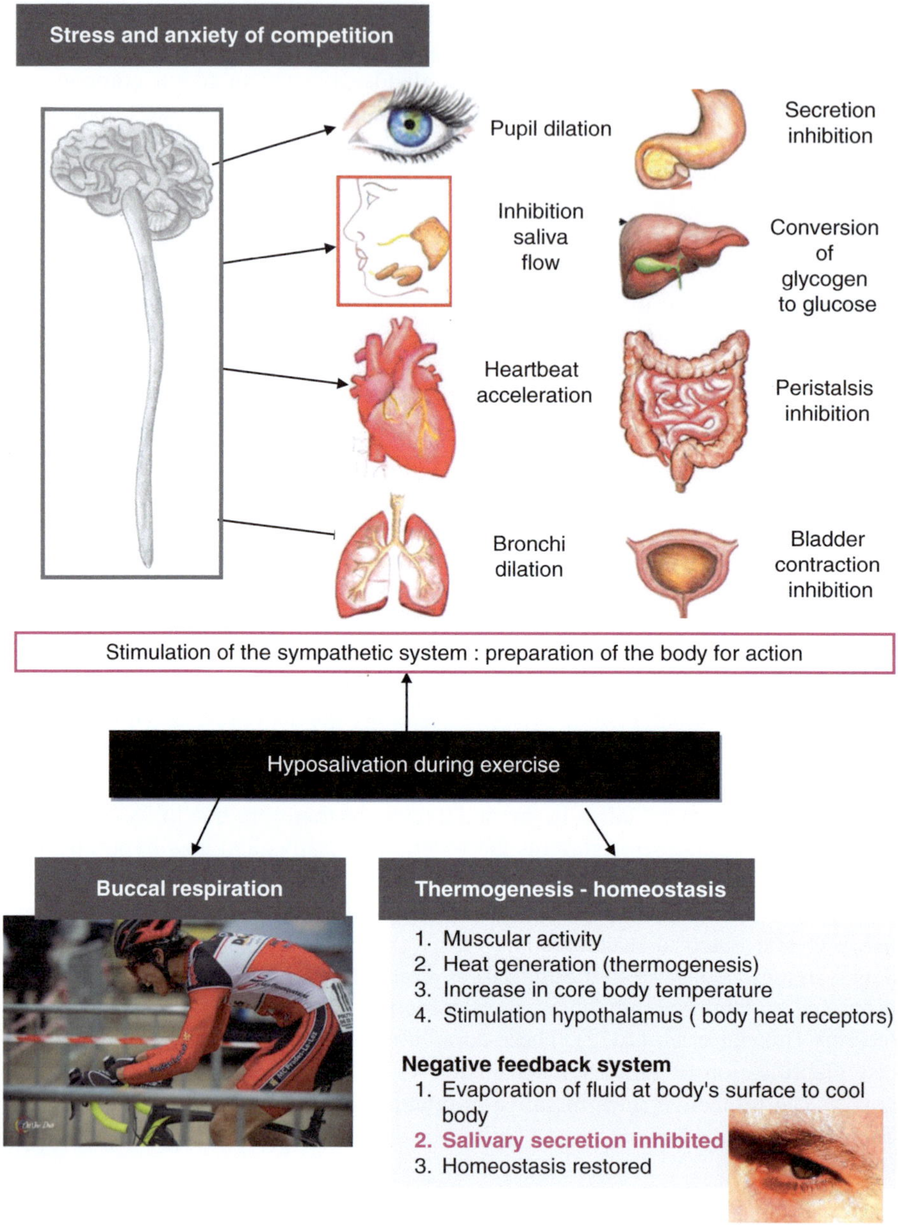

Fig. 8.2 The causes of hyposalivation during exercise

Table 8.1 The roles and mechanisms of saliva action on oral health

Role	Mechanism of protection
Lubrication	Enables deglutition – phonation
Antibacterial (caries)	(a) Inhibition of bacterial adhesion to dental surfaces (b) Salivary buffer capacity (remineralisation)
Protection against acidic dissolution of dental surfaces	(a) Inhibition of adhesion of acidic alimentation onto the tooth's surface (b) Selectively permeable layer and buffering action of its bicarbonate content (c) Flushing action on acids (d) Remineralisation: inorganic constituents Ca^{2+}, PO_4^{2-}, and F^- slow dissolution and facilitate remineralisation
Immunity	Presence of immunoglobulins, lysozymes, mucines and antimicrobial peptides

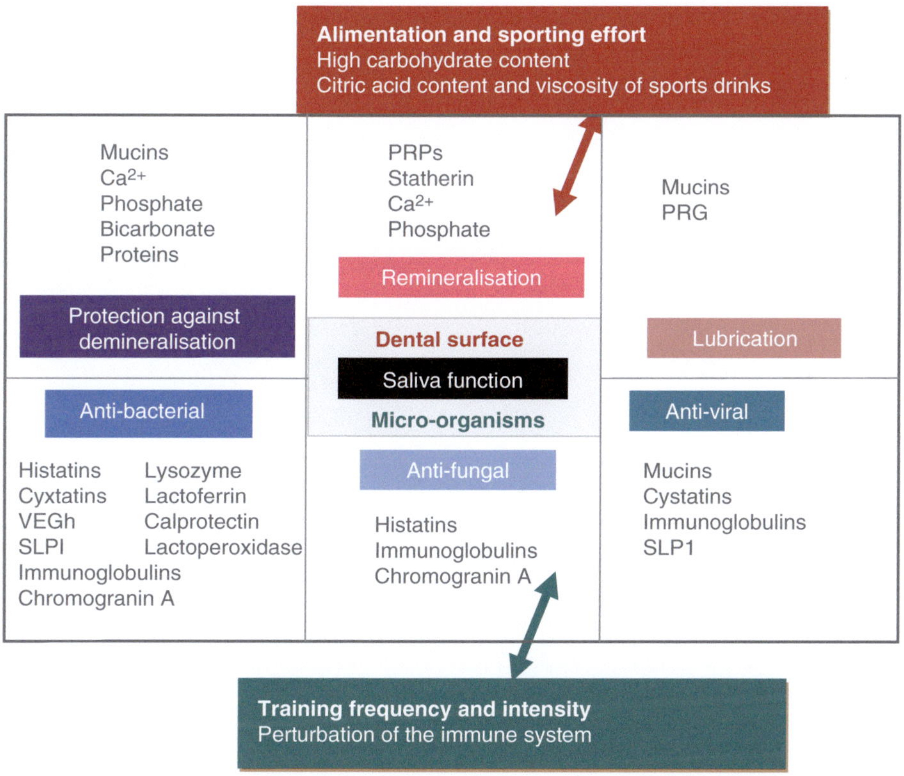

Fig. 8.3 The connection between hyposalivation in sport, demineralisation of dental surfaces and oral infections

References

Buzalaf M, Rabelo A, Reis Hannas A, Thiemi KM (2012) Saliva and dental erosion. J Appl Oral Sci 20:493–502

Dawes C (1987) Physiological factors affecting salivary flow rate, oral sugar clearance, and the sensation of dry mouth in man. J Dent Res 66:648–653

Gonsalez S, Sung H (2014) Oral manifestations and their treatment in Sjögren's syndrome. Oral Dis 20(2):153–161

Lamendin H (2004) Odontologie du Sport. CdP, Rueil-Malmaison

Levine MJ (1993) Salivary macromolecules. A structure/function synopsis. Ann N Y Acad Sci 694:11–16

Li T-L, Gleeson M (2004) The effect of single and repeated bouts of prolonged cycling and circadian variation on saliva flow rate, immunoglobulin A and alpha-amylase responses. J Sports Sci 22(11–12):1015–1024

Mandel ID (1989) The role of saliva in maintaining oral homeostasis. J Am Dent Assoc 119:298–304

Turner JR, Hiroshi S (2002) Understanding salivary fluid and protein secretion. Oral Dis 8:3–11

Oral Health Risk Factor: Psychology of the Athlete

9

9.1 Introduction

Psychological traits of athletes are less conspicuous oral health risks in sport but, nevertheless, can be responsible for specific problems of the oral cavity. The first risk is stress and anxiety, linked to athletic performance and competition. The second risk is body image and the higher probability of eating disorders amongst certain athletic populations.

Stress is commonly associated to bruxism, which is notoriously difficult to treat. Not only does it affect the oral cavity but also the craniofacial sphere and can have systemised repercussions on posture and biomechanics, provoking injury.

Unfortunately, body dissatisfaction is common amongst women in Western society. Athletes are particularly at risk from eating disorders due to the added pressure of performance in their chosen sport. With anorexia and bulimia nervosa cases particularly high in certain disciplines, oral complications are frequent. Several domains of dental practice are implied. Therapeutic solutions address dental caries and erosion, xerostomia, periodontal disease and even temporomandibular disorders.

9.2 The First Risk: Stress and Anxiety

According to the European Agency for Safety and Health at Work (2015), stress is the incapacity to deal with certain situations: ‘Stress is experienced when an individual feels an imbalance between what is required of them and their ability to deal with the situation. Although stress is perceived psychologically, it can also affect physical health. Stress becomes a risk to health and safety when perpetuating over time’.

With increasingly fast-paced lifestyles, participation in sport is frequently advocated as a natural stress reliever. Aerobic exercise sustained for 30 minutes or more releases endorphins ‘happy hormones’, giving a sensation of wellbeing and increased morale. Sport permits the individual to evacuate tension and canalise energy, hence placing a perspective on everyday problems.

S.C. Budd, J.-C. Egea, *Sport and Oral Health*, DOI 10.1007/978-3-319-53423-7_9

9.2.1 Stress, Athletes and Sport

Paradoxically, sport can also become a source of stress. If too much emphasis is placed upon physical improvement and winning, it can become a constraint rather than a pleasure. Furthermore, competition-related stress may prove to be too much for certain individuals. In the realm of sports psychology, anxiety disorders are well documented amongst both male and female athletes (Hoyer and Kleinert 2010). At elite level, athletes are subjected to intense mental and social stress. It is often assumed that to perform at such a high level, the athlete must be psychologically sound. Unfortunately, this is not always the case (Markser 2011).

According to Kerdijk et al. 2016, perhaps unsurprisingly, team athletes felt most stress when in competition as opposed to training. in other words, in a situation of threat. A combination of factors will determine how an athlete reacts to this stress. Influential factors include personality, gender, the type of sport played and environmental factors such as the social context (Markser 2011). The coping strategy of the athlete will also depend upon the perception of the stressful situation as a threat or a challenge. Figure 9.1 based on Kerdijk et al. (2016) and DeLongis and Holtzman (2005) neatly summarises several notions of sports psychology and stress in sport.

So how does stress in sport pose a risk to athletic patients in the field of dentistry?

9.2.2 Stress and Anxiety as a Risk Factor to Oral Health: Bruxism

A likely psychosomatic expression of stress in dentistry is bruxism. It is defined as a diurnal or nocturnal parafunctional activity that includes clenching, bracing,

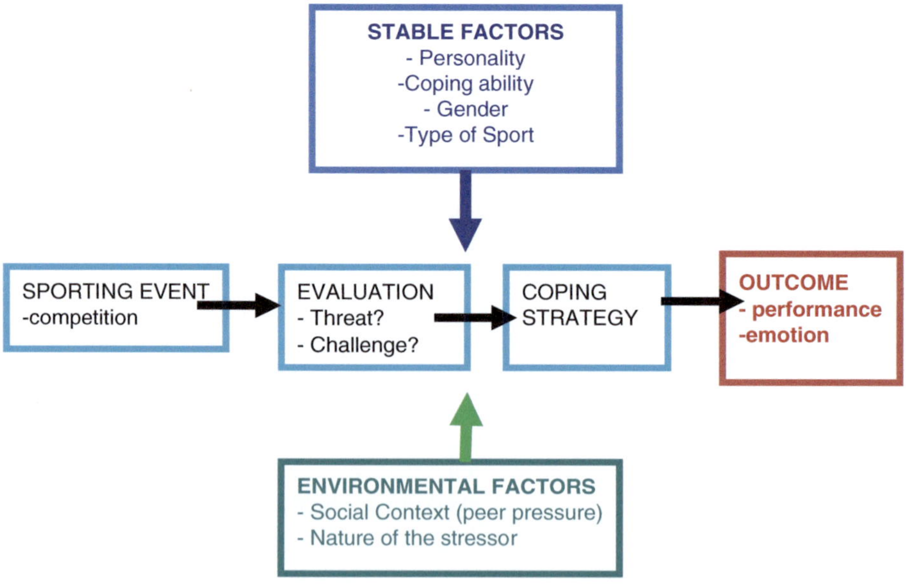

Fig. 9.1 Stress, athletes and performance

gnashing and grinding of teeth, which affects approximately 20% of the population. Although the aetiology of bruxism is multifactorial, it is believed to be associated to stress (Lavigne et al. 2008). Furthermore, athletes participating in strenuous sporting activities often clench their jaws during maximal effort. A questionnaire distributed to a British Athletics Club, Blackheath Harriers, revealed that nearly 40% of runners reported this form of centric bruxism whilst competing in competitions or during intense training sessions. This percentage is double that of the general population.

9.2.3 Repercussions of Bruxism on Oral and General Health

Repercussions on the oral cavity are numerous. Restoration is difficult, and effective treatment requires a collaboration of different branches of health professions. Immediate symptoms observed in dentistry include dental hypersensitivity, attrition, fractures, loss of the vertical dimension, cheek and tongue biting, gingival recession and the destruction of ceramic prosthodontics. Unfortunately, if left untreated, consequences of bruxism can extend beyond the oral cavity and ultimately interfere with athletic performance. As with problems of dental occlusion and infection, it is important to recognise the connections between the oral cavity and the rest of the body. Figure 9.2 lists the consequences of bruxism. They can affect the oral cavity, the orofacial and craniofacial spheres, or even induce secondary symptoms elsewhere. Photos in Fig. 9.3 show the reality of these consequences – both on hard dental tissue and facial muscles.

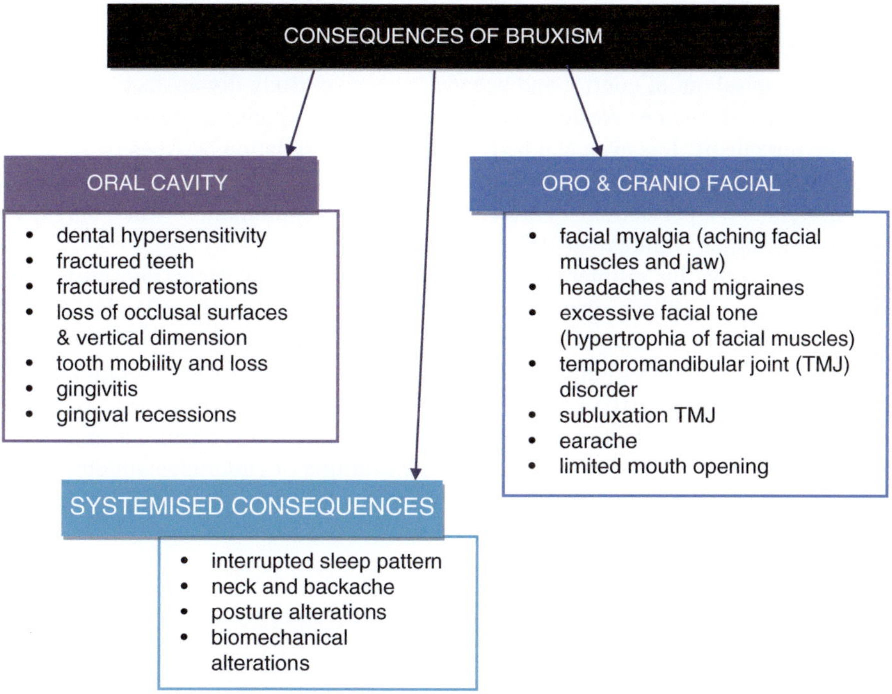

Fig. 9.2 Oral and general health consequences of bruxism

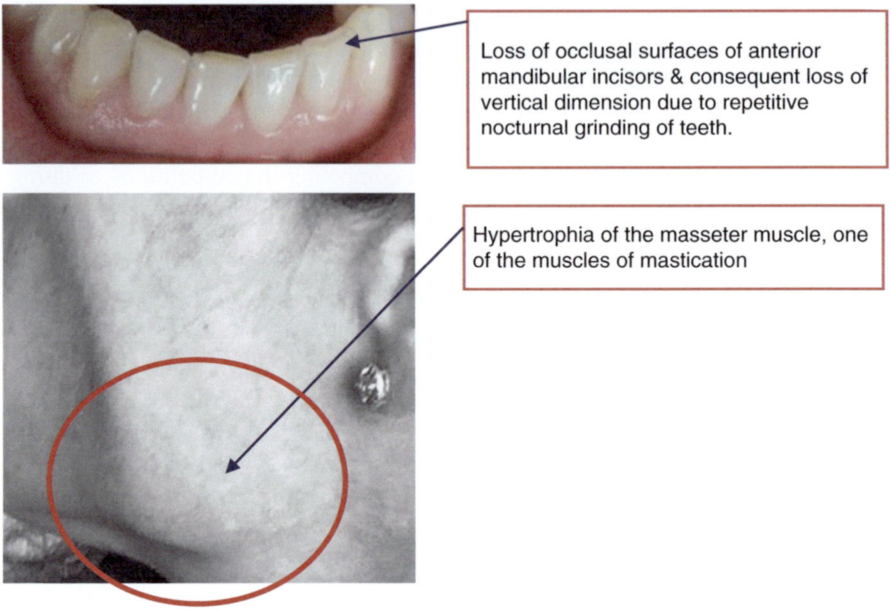

Fig. 9.3 Consequences of bruxism: high-level endurance athlete

9.3 The Second Risk: Body Image

A great incentive of many people to exercise and participate in sport is to lose weight. What starts as good intentions, such as eating healthily and doing exercise, can easily spiral out of control and become excessive. Body dissatisfaction is common amongst women in Western society, as the 'perfect body' associated to beauty is often unrealistic. It is even claimed that there is a correlation between being slim, social success and admiration (Guillemot and Lanexaire 1997). This, coupled with low esteem and a perfectionist nature, is a dangerous combination which may lead to eating disorders (Lindeman 1994).

Unfortunately, this problematic is accentuated in athletes. Here, the sportsman/woman may wish to lose weight, not just to be more 'physically attractive' but to improve performance. Leanness is related to performance for obvious physiological reasons. Athletes who weigh more than their optimum performance weight are at a disadvantage (Currie 2010).

Interestingly, the 'ideal' morphology to which athletes may aspire is similar to the western concept of beauty. If we take the example of endurance athletes, high jumpers and well-known supermodels, they are tall, lean and well-toned, the western ideal.

9.3.1 Eating Disorders: Anorexia Nervosa and Bulimia Nervosa, Prevalence in Sport

The two most common eating disorders which may result are anorexia nervosa and bulimia nervosa. Anorexia nervosa is characterised by a refusal to eat. Bulimia nervosa is characterised by binge eating, accompanied by vomiting or laxative usage. Although eating disorders are common in adolescents and young adults, studies have found a higher incidence amongst athletes than the general population. On average 13.5% of athletes fall victim – 20.1% female and 7.7% male (Sundgot-Borgen and Klungland 2004).

Athletes participating in disciplines where weight is prerequisite to performance are particularly at risk. For example, high incidences of eating disorders were documented in a British study on female distance runners, in which 29 out of 184 female athletes (16%) were diagnosed with an eating disorder of clinical severity (Hulley and Hill 2001). Equally, athletes in aesthetic sports are vulnerable. A study on Norwegian gymnasts stated that 42% of their female athletes suffered from an eating disorder, despite being classified as normal weight (Sundgot-Borgen and Klungland 2004).

9.3.2 Eating Disorders and Oral Health

Unfortunately, the psychological and physiological repercussions of chronic eating disorders may, in extreme cases, have fatal outcomes such as cardiac arrest or suicide. In dentistry, the practitioner's role is not only to treat the symptoms but also to play a potentially vital role in the detection of the illness and consequent referral to medical specialists.

Table 9.1 summarises these oral complications found in such patients (Little 2002, Johansson et al. 2010 and Keller et al. 2012). Comparing the two eating disorders, bulimia nervosa is the most destructive – unfortunately all aspects of oral

Table 9.1 Oral complications of anorexia nervosa and bulimia nervosa

Oral complication	Anorexia nervosa	Bulimia nervosa
Dental erosion	No	Yes
Tooth sensitivity	No	Yes
Xerostomia	Yes	Yes/No
Dry mouth (complaint)	Yes	Yes
Dental caries	No	Yes
Periodontal disease	No	Yes
Enlarged parotid glands	Yes	Yes
Atrophic mucosa	Yes	No
Poor oral hygiene	No	Yes
Temporomandibular disorders	No	Yes
Craniofacial disorders	No	Yes

health are implicated. A patient may present a few or several of the following oral consequences:

The photos in Fig. 9.4, courtesy of Dr. Christel Dessalces Olenisac, illustrate these dental repercussions, affecting hard and soft tissues alike.

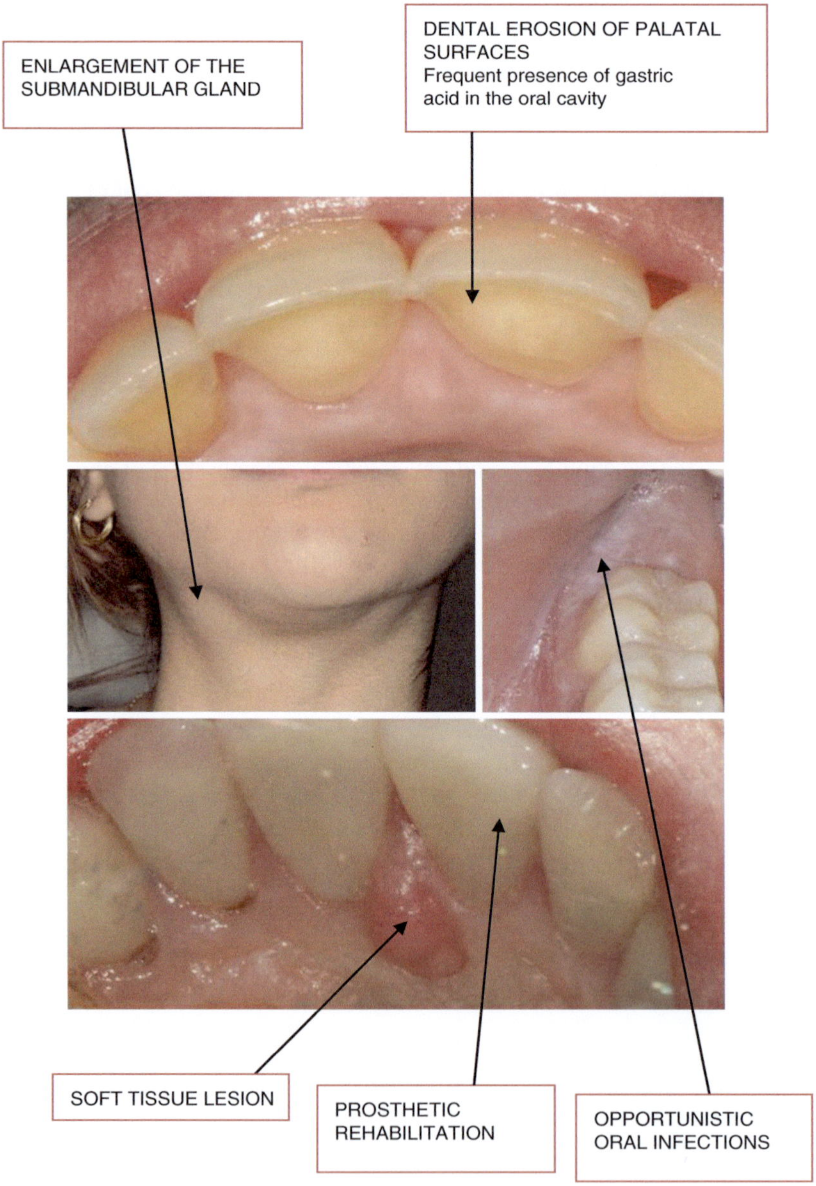

Fig. 9.4 Oral complications of anorexia and bulimia nervosa, images courtesy of Dr. Christel Dessalces Olenisac

Interestingly, a study by Sirin et al. (2011) claimed that sufferers of eating disorders also exhibited most fear when undergoing basic oral procedures at the dental surgery.

References

Currie A (2010) Sport and eating disorders – understanding and managing the risks. Asian J Sports Med 1:63–68

DeLongis A, Holtzman S (2005) Coping in context: the role of stress, social support, and personality in coping. J Pers 73:1633–1656

European Agency for Safety and Health At Work (2015) Un guide électronique pratique pour gérer les risques psychosociaux. https://www.healthy-workplaces.eu/fr/tools-and-resources/a-guide-to-psychosocial-risks. Accessed 10 Feb 2016

Guillemot A, Lanexaire M (1997) Anorexie mentale et boulimie: le poids de la culture, 2nd edn. Masson, Paris

Hoyer J, Kleinert J (2010) Lesitungssport und psychische Strorungen. Psychotherapeutenjournal 3:252–260

Hulley AJ, Hill AJ (2001) Eating disorders and health in elite women distance runners. Int J Eat Disord 30:312–317

Johansson AK, Johansson A, Unell L, Norring C, Carlsson GE (2010) Eating disorders and signs and symptoms of temporomandibular disorders, a matched case-control study. Swed Dent J 34(3): 139–147

Keller EE, Baltali E, Liang X, Zhao K, Huebner M, Kai-Nan A (2012) Temporomandibular custom hemijoint replacement prosthesis: prospective clinical and kinematic study. J Oral Maxillofac Surg (Off J Am Assoc Oral Maxillofac Surg) 70(2):276–288

Kerdijk C, van der Kamp J, Polman R (2016) The influence of the social environment context in stress and coping in sport. Front Psychol 7:875

Lavigne GJ, KhourY S et al (2008) Bruxism physiology and pathology: an overview for clinicians. J Oral Rehabil 35:476–494

Lindeman AK (1994) Self-esteem: its application to eating disorders and athletes. Int J Sport Nutr 4:237–252

Little JW (2002) Eating disorders: dental implications. Oral Surge Oral Med Oral Pathol Oral Radiol Endod 93:138–143

Markser VZ (2011) Sport psychiatry and psychotherapy. Mental strains and disorders in professional sports. Challenge and answer to societal changes. Eur Arch Psychiatry Clin Neurosci 261(Suppl 2):182–185

Sundgot-Borgen J, Klungland TM (2004) Prevalence of eating disorders in elite athletes is higher than in the general population. ClinJ Sport Med (OffJ Can Acad Sport Med) 14:25–32

Sirin Y, Yucel B, Firat D, Husseinova-Sen S (2011) Assessment of dental fear and anxiety levels in eating disorder patients undergoing minor oral surgery. J Oral Maxillofac Surg (OffJ Am Assoc Oral Maxillofac Surg) 69:2078–2085

Oral Health Risk Factor: Dental Traumatology in Sport

10

10.1 Introduction

Traumatic dental and maxillofacial injuries are an everyday reality. Globally, 20–30% of permanent dentition is affected, with sporting activity for children and young adolescents being the main culprit. With an increasing popularity of organised sporting events for youths, dental and facial injuries have become regular occurrences.

Numerous factors predispose certain athletes to certain types of orofacial sports-related traumatology. For example, the type of physical exertion required, whether explosive or sustained, influences the athlete's corporal position and vulnerability to very different dental lesions. Equally, if the sport has a high probability of contact, either with other players or equipment, the athlete is obviously at greater risk. Interestingly, the characteristics of the athlete himself are also important considerations and include his or her oral physiology, behaviour during play and level of participation.

Reducing the risk of orofacial traumatology in sport is an important issue for dental practitioners, athletes and their coaches. Prophylactic measures are indispensable to prevent potentially serious consequences (Fig. 10.1).

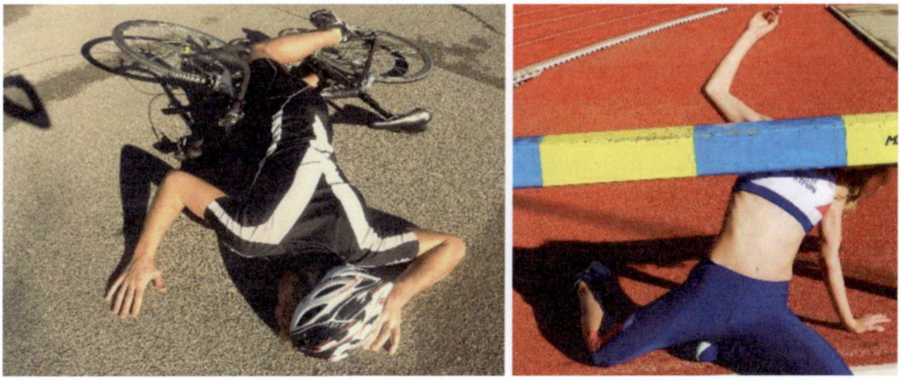

Fig. 10.1 Dental traumatology: a risk in all sports

S.C. Budd, J.-C. Egea, *Sport and Oral Health*, DOI 10.1007/978-3-319-53423-7_10

10.2 The Prevalence of Orofacial Sports-Related Trauma in America

Over the last 10 years, it is estimated that 46 million young Americans annually participated in sport, of which 30 million in organised competitive events (Barron and Powell 2005). With such high numbers taking part, prevention rather than cure is of utmost importance (Bourguignon and Sigurdsson 2009). Amongst youths, two of the most risky sports in America are basketball and baseball. They have been reported to have the highest prevalence of dental trauma in sport amongst children aged 7–17 (Kumamoto and Yoshinobu 2004). Given orofacial sports-related injuries occur during both organised athletic events and unorganised recreational activities, incidence data on sports injuries is likely to be under-reported (Ranalli 2002).

10.3 Maxillofacial Positions and Dental Traumatology

During physical exertion, a given athlete adopts one of two different maxillofacial positions, depending on the type of exercise undertaken. Each of these positions renders the athlete vulnerable to two different forms of orofacial injury. Let us compare sustained effort and explosive effort.

10.3.1 Prolonged Aerobic Exercise

During prolonged effort, typical of endurance sports, nasal breathing transforms into buccal breathing. The body's position is one of extension, the position of rest. The athlete is vulnerable to extended corporal injuries. These include lesions of the temporomandibular joint (TMJ), rachidian vertebrae and cerebral injuries, equivalent to whiplash in a car accident.

10.3.2 Explosive Anaerobic Exercise

Alternatively, in more explosive team sports, an athlete often clenches his/her jaws. This recruits the facial muscles in a protective stance. This second form of trauma is more localised. The athlete is more likely to suffer soft tissue lesions or dental or mandibular fractures at high impact.

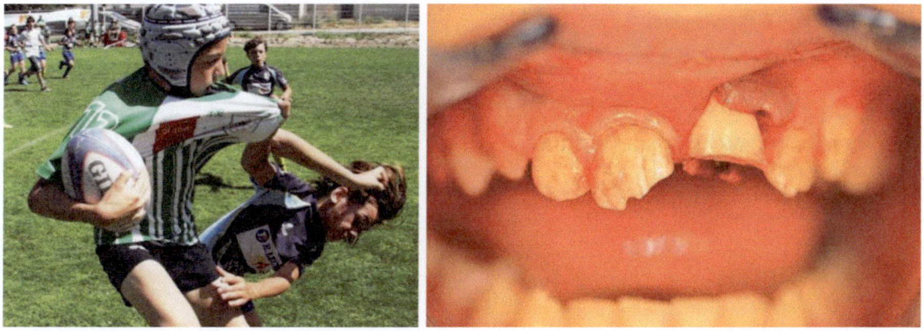

Fig. 10.2 Dental traumatology in sport: incisors at risk

Dental or maxillofacial traumatology is a true emergency for the dentist. Such sports-related injuries involve predominantly the upper lip, maxilla and maxillary incisors. Permanent maxillary incisors are particularly affected and account for at least 50% of all dental traumas (Martin et al. 1990, Kumamoto and Yoshinobu 2004; Glendor 2009) (Fig. 10.2).

10.4 Which Sports Pose the Greatest Risk?

Sports with a high probability of falls or contact with players or other equipment pose the greatest threat. Obvious culprits include boxing, ice hockey and rugby. In addition, perhaps surprisingly, several endurance sports have been considered in scientific literature as high risk. Examples include cycling, skiing and swimming (Emshoff et al. 1997 and Levin et al. 2003). A review study by Kumamoto et al. (2004) revealed that 85 million Americans cycle every year. Of these, 540 000 are victims of orofacial trauma. With regard to dental traumatology in sport, the International Dental Federation (FDI) categorised certain sports as either being high risk or medium risk (World Dental Federation 1990) (Fig. 10.3).

To help combat the risk of orofacial injury, the American Dental Association recommends the usage of mouthguards in the majority of the sports listed in Fig. 10.2. A multitude of sports are implied, including less obvious disciplines such as weightlifting or shot putting.

HIGH RISK

- Team sports with rough contact and accessories

- Sports requiring good balance

EXAMPLES

American football
Hockey
Ice hockey
Lacrosse
Martial Arts
Rugby
Skating
Skateboarding
Mountain biking

MEDIUM RISK

- Team sports with less contact, but risk of contact or falling

EXAMPLES

Football
Handball
Basketball
Diving
Racquet sports
Diving
Parachuting
Waterpolo

Fig. 10.3 Orofacial traumatology: high- and medium-risk sports

10.5 Which Athletes Are at Greatest Risk?

Many criteria determine the vulnerability of athletes to orofacial injury. The type of sport played is just one determinant. Other factors predisposing athletes to traumatic dental injuries in sport include the characteristics of the athlete himself, environmental factors and the type of participation in a given sport (Glendor 2009). An athlete's oral disposition, dental overjet and inadequate lip coverage have been considered a major risk factor for many years (Burden 1995). In addition, behavioural tendencies during play are also to be considered. Lalloo et al. (2003) claim hyperactive children are particularly vulnerable.

With regard to environmental factors, demographic information, attitudes of coaches and the general organisation of the given sport influence the risk of accidents (American Academy of Pediatric Dentistry 2013).

A third major theme is participation. Participation entails the intensity, level played and whether it is a training session or competition. For example, several studies have concluded that professional players are at a lower risk of dental trauma during play (Mourouzis and Koumoura 2005). They are more likely to use preventive measures such as mouthguards and master gestures during play. Figure 10.4 recapitulates the factors that influence an individual's risk to orofacial traumatic injuries in sport.

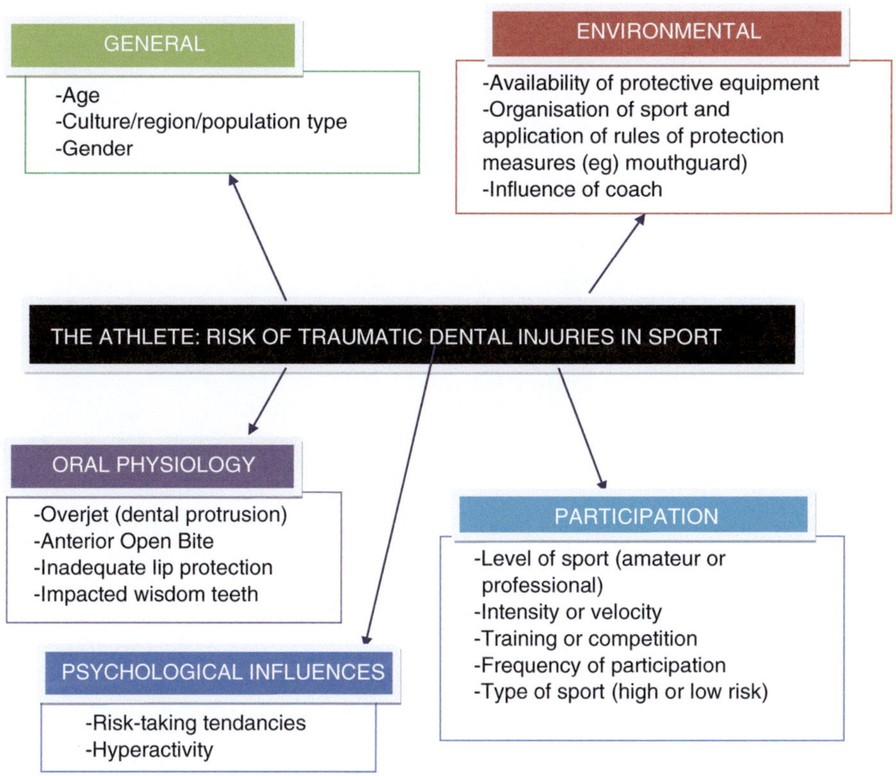

Fig. 10.4 Factors predisposing athletes to dental trauma in sport

10.6 Reducing the Risk of Orofacial Traumatology in Sport

Given the consequences of orofacial trauma, which include pain, psychological repercussions, the interruption of training and certain economic implications, prevention is paramount.

The role of orofacial protective measures cannot be underestimated (Fig. 10.5). For example, a study on the incidence of orofacial trauma in American football dropped from 50% to under 1% in a study by Knapik et al. (2007) when facemasks and mouthguards were enforced. Equally, Ferrari et al. (2002) investigated hockey players. They found a particularly low incidence of oral trauma in this high-contact sport, partially thanks to the increased usage of mouthguards in the sport. Research suggests that many sports that do not formally require mouthguards should encourage male and female participants to use orofacial protectors, even if not compulsory for play (Kumamoto and Yoshinobu 2004).

The role of the dental practitioner is multifaceted. They must inform and educate athletes of all ages of the potential risk of their chosen sport. They must be able to

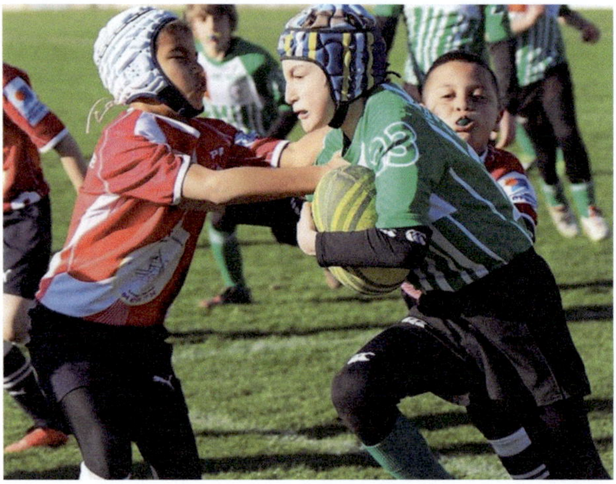

Fig. 10.5 Preventing orofacial traumatology in sport: the use of mouthguards

clinically evaluate the individual predisposition of the patient to sports-related oral traumatology and to be capable of providing a clinically adapted solution.

References

American Academy of Pediatric Dentistry (2013) Policy on prevention of sports related orofacial injuries. Oral Health Policies 37:71–75

Barron M, Powell J (2005) Fundamentals of injury prevention in youth sports. J Pediatr Dent Care 11(2):10–12

Bourguignon C, Sigurdsson A (2009) Preventive strategies for traumatic dental injuries. Dent Clin N Am 53:729–749

Burden DJ (1995) An investigation of the association between overjet size, lip coverage, and traumatic injury to maxillary incisors. Eur J Orthod 17:513–517

Emshoff R, Schöning H, Röthler G, Waldhart E (1997) Trends in the incidence and cause of sport-related mandibular fractures: a retrospective analysis. J Oral Maxillofac Surg (Official J Am Assoc Oral Maxillofac Surg) 55:585–592

Ferrari CH, Ferreria de Mederios JM (2002) Dental trauma and level of information: mouthguard use in different contact sports. Dent Traumatol (Off Publ Int Assoc Dent Traumatol) 18:144–147

Glendor U (2009) Aaetiology and risk factors related to traumatic dental injuries-a review of the literature. Dent Traumatol (Official Publ Int Assoc Dent Traumatol) 25:19–31

Knapik JJ, Marshall SW, Lee RB, Darakjy SS, Jones SB, Mitchener TA, delaCruz GG, Jones BH (2007) Mouthguards in sport activities: history, physical properties and injury prevention effectiveness. Sports Med (Auckland, N.Z.) 37:117–144

Kumamoto DP, Yoshinobu M (2004) A literature review of sports related orofacial trauma. Gen Dent 52:270–280

Lalloo R (2003) Risk factors for major injuries to the face and teeth. Dent Traumatol 19:12–14

Levin L, Friedlander LD, Geiger SB (2003) Dental and oral trauma and mouthguard use during sport activities in Israel. Dent Traumatol (Off Publ Int Assoc Dent Traumatol) 19:237–242

Martin IG, Daly CG, Liew VP (1990) After-hours treatment of anterior dental trauma in Newcastle and western Sydney: a four-year study. Aust Dent J 35:27–31

Mourouzis C, Koumoura F (2005) Sports related maxillofacial fractures: a retrospective study of 125 patients. Int J Oral Maxillofac Surg 34:635–638

Ranalli D (2002) Sports dentistry and dental traumatology. Dent Traumatol (Off Publ Int Assoc Dent Traumatol) 18:231–236

World Dental Federation. Commission on dental products. 1990

Other Sports-Related Oral Health Risk Factors: Medication, Education and Access to Dental Care

11

11.1 Introduction

Self-medication and doping in athletes, education, knowledge, motivation and access to dental care are important risk factors that can affect the oral health of active patients.

Athletes have a tendency to self-medicate. Injuries are frequent, especially those of an inflammatory nature. Doping also exists, and the dental practitioner must take care not to prescribe common molecules that may give a positive result in a doping control.

The prioritisation of oral care amongst athletes is a further relevant consideration. A myriad of factors influence the place of oral health on an athlete's list of prerogatives, including a host of external influences such as education and marketing of dental issues. The athlete's interpretation of this information will determine the significance of personal oral care. A final problem is access to dental care. Elite athletes away on training camps are particularly at risk, as are athletes who live in disadvantaged areas.

11.2 Athletes and Medication

It is easy to assume that athletic patients in good health would not need to use prescribed medication nor indulge in excess consumption when necessary. This relationship is not straightforward. Injuries are common in sport, and the 'will to improve' may tempt the athlete to self-medicate and take supplements.

11.2.1 Self-Medication and Athletes

Athletes of all levels may self-medicate either to relieve injury symptoms or to improve performance. Muscular and tendon pains are particularly frequent in athletes. A common reflex is to 'see if it clears up' with a few days' rest and to take a

S.C. Budd, J.-C. Egea, *Sport and Oral Health*, DOI 10.1007/978-3-319-53423-7_11

couple of over-the-counter antalgics or anti-inflammatories. Alternatively, the desire to improve performance may tempt athletes to take a variety of supplements.

For example, at elite level, a study of the 2000 Sydney Olympics revealed a dangerous overuse of nonsteroidal anti-inflammatory drugs (NSAIDs), with athletes taking several different molecules at the same time. They were therefore subjected to an increased risk of medication interactions (Corrigan and Rymantas 2003).

The practitioner must therefore inform himself on any medication taken for sporting reasons, to avoid such interactions and surcharges of a given medication.

11.2.2 Doping and Athletes

It would be naive to assume an athlete wouldn't indulge in doping. Currently, the president of the International Olympic Committee, Sebastian Coe, is on a mission to expose the extent of doping in sport. The dentist must appreciate that a given athlete could be abusing banned substances to improve performance. The more intensive the training schedule, the greater the risk. Inversely, they must also be aware that what they prescribe could be classified as a doping agent.

11.3 Education, Knowledge and Motivation: Risk Factor

Oral health behaviour and prioritisation are influenced by a variety of factors, such as family, upbringing, access to treatment and peers. For athletes, it is also very likely to be influenced by fellow athletes, sports coaches, support staff and organisations (Needleman et al. 2015). Figure 11.1 recapitulates the influencing environmental factors and personal considerations which decide the importance of oral health for a given individual.

Paradoxically, elite athletes often have little knowledge or prioritisation of their oral health, despite fine tuning of their bodies to optimal performance.

In France, children and adolescents are invited to have regular dental controls which are free of charge. The encouragement of athletes to visit their dentist by influential acquaintances, such as the sports trainer or doctor, would undoubtably help prioritise oral health in the sporting world.

The technique employed by their dentist to inform, motivate without blame (Yevlahova and Satur 2009) and educate plays a part, though oral health professionals alone are unlikely to achieve sustained improvements. Working in collaborative partnerships with other relevant professionals and agencies is more likely to educate and motivate both athletes and the general population (Watt 2002).

11.4 Complicated Access to Dental Treatment: Risk Factor

This section applies principally to elite athletes. They train several times a day, are often away from home and may spend many months of the year in rural training camps. The schedule of the elite athlete is therefore complicated, and access to

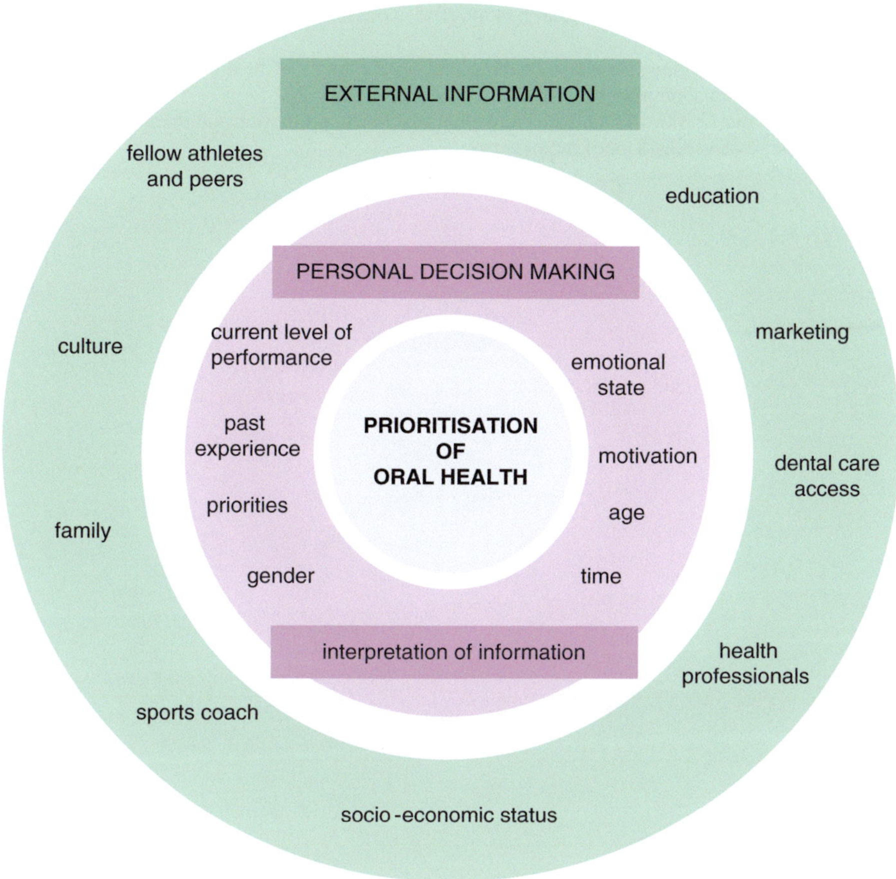

Fig. 11.1 Factors influencing athletes' prioritisation of oral health

dental care is limited. It is therefore important to adapt to their intensive programme and insist on the importance of prophylactic measures.

Athletes living in disadvantaged areas that lack dental care infrastructure are also at risk from oral health problems. Again, prevention is the key and programmed check-ups will help avoid more serious complications.

Recent advances in Internet technology have permitted the development of a new form of prevention in oral care, known as 'telemedicine'. Using oral cameras, the patient can film his oral cavity, providing the dentist with an initial global overview of his oral health. It is an efficient and comfortable form of consultation, though it does not replace a clinical exam.

References

Corrigan B, Rymantas K (2003) Medication use in athletes selected for doping control at the Sydney Olympics 2000. Clin J Sport Med (Off J Can Acad Sport Med) 13:33–40

Needleman I, Ashley P, Fine P, Haddad F et al (2015) Oral health and elite sport performance. Br J Sports Med 49:3–6
Watt RG (2002) Emerging theories into the social determinants of health: implications for oral health promotion. Community Dent Oral Epidemiol 30:241–247
Yevlahova D, Satur J (2009) Models for individual oral health promotion and their effectiveness: a systematic review. Aust Dent J 54:190–197

Part III

Clinical Reality: Physiological Processes and Oral Health

An explanation of the biological phenomena threatening the oral cavity and beyond and how athletic performance is interlinked with oral health.

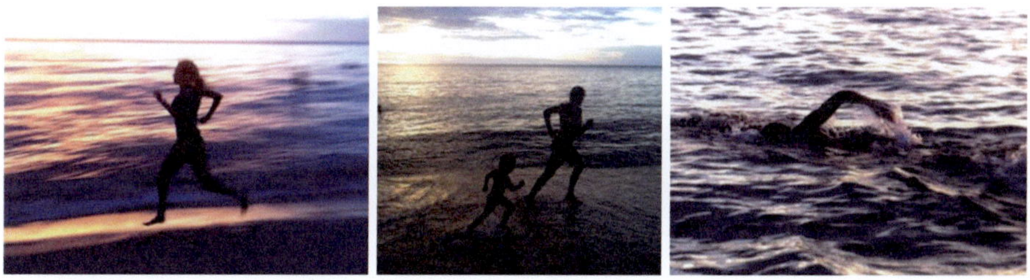

Sport, Periodontal Consequences and Athletic Patients

12

12.1 Introduction

Gingivitis and periodontitis are two of the most common infections to inflict humans. Athletes are exposed to the same risk factors as their sedentary counterparts for developing periodontal disease. These include dental calculus, bad hygiene, unfavourable dental anatomy, modification of systemic factors such as the immune or endocrine system or even medication taken.

However, periodontal examinations carried out on the London Olympians by Needleman et al. (2013) revealed a catastrophic prevalence of reversible gingivitis amongst athletes (75%), with 15% suffering from irreversible periodontitis. This high presence of gingivitis, which, in the majority of cases, is caused by dental plaque, suggests that oral hygiene was not high on the priority list of physical health of these Olympic athletes.

Equally, a cross-sectional study of athletes that participated in the 2011 Nigerian University Games revealed that 36.3% had gingival bleeding yet only 40% had ever been to the dentist (Azodo and Osazuwa 2013).

Furthermore, studies have revealed specific periodontal diseases that have a particularly high incidence amongst athletes. Three different periodontal consequences are investigated: firstly, precocious alveolysis, exacerbated by neglected oral hygiene and a modulation of the immune system; secondly, gingival hypertrophy associated to anabolic steroid use; and finally, swimmers' calculus, a form of dental plaque which is linked to frequent training in swimming pools.

12.2 Specific Case: Precocious Alveolysis

Loss of alveolar bone over time is an inevitable consequence of aging. In a healthy individual, this process normally starts around the age of 35, known as adult periodontitis, and progresses slowly with no defects in the host's defence system (American Academy of Periodontology 1989; Wiebe and Putnins 2000).

S.C. Budd, J.-C. Egea, *Sport and Oral Health*, DOI 10.1007/978-3-319-53423-7_12

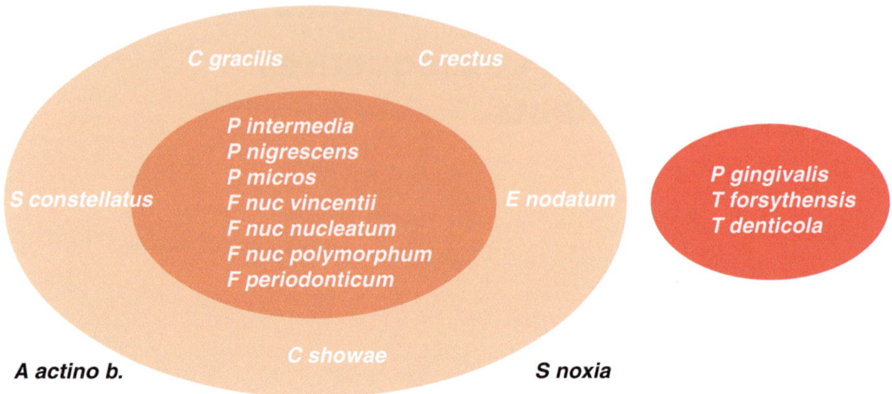

Fig. 12.1 The complexes of anaerobic bacteria common to periodontitis based on Socransky's classification

However, studies by Lamendin and Tavernier, dating back as early as the 1970s, described the phenomenon of precocious alveolysis. Initially found in young Russian soldiers aged 20 to 30, they discovered the same plight in high-level amateur athletes, aged between 18 and 30 (Lamendin 1983, 2004; Lamendin and Tavernier 2008).

Precocious alveolysis, a form of periodontitis, is an inflammatory disease which forms periodontal pockets. Here it is responsible for a *premature* loss of the supporting tissues of teeth, the periodontium. The destructive action of specific anaerobic bacteria results in the progressive destruction of the periodontal ligament and alveolar bone. Clinical observation distinguishes gingivitis from periodontitis by the loss of periodontal attachments.

The bacteria responsible for this premature loss of alveolar bone belong to distinct bacterial complexes found in subgingival plaque, as classified by Socransky et al. (1998). The anaerobic culprits are *Actinobacillus actinomycetemcomitans* and those classified in the red and orange complexes shown in Fig. 12.1, in particular *Prevotella intermedia* and *Porphyromonas gingivalis.*

12.2.1 Why Are Athletes at Risk of Precocious Alveolysis?

Generally speaking, an individual becomes more vulnerable to periodontal disease if subject to bad oral hygiene and a diversity of risk factors including bacterial interactions and an impaired host – response system.

Socransky et al. (1998) identified four factors necessary for periodontal tissue destruction:

1. The presence of anaerobic pathogenic bacteria, Gram –
2. The absence of protective bacteria, Gram +

3. An immune system deficiency
4. Unfavourable oral environment (bad oral hygiene, stress)

Athletes may therefore be particularly susceptible if suffering from a weaker immune system linked to overtraining, coupled to an unfavourable oral environment. Another influential factor is undoubtedly that of hyposalivation associated to intensive, prolonged sporting effort, hence a diminution of the protective factors saliva provides the buccal cavity.

Interestingly, this phenomenon has also been associated to drug addicts and has been found in athletes participating in sports where doping is rife (Lamendin and Tavernier 2008).

12.3 Gingival Hypertrophy

An interesting study by Ozcelik et al. (2006) investigated the correlation between anabolic androgenic steroid (AAS) abuse and gingival enlargement, on a group of 24 bodybuilders.

The results showed that the AAS abusers had statistically higher scores of gingival thickness, extent of gingival encroachment and total gingival enlargement scores ($P < 0.001$ each) compared to non-users.

The use of anabolic steroids is generally associated to explosive sports, with oxygen-boosting drugs such as erythropoietin (EPO) more commonly linked to endurance events. However, these anabolic steroids facilitate many aspects of training, even in long-distance sports. Athletes who misuse these substances are able to train harder and for longer, recover faster from exertion and improve their muscular efficiency and, indirectly, their VO2 max. We need only to look at Mathew Kisorio, the third fastest half-marathoner in history, tested positive for anabolic steroids during the 2012 Kenyan Track and Field Championships.

12.4 Swimmers' Calculus

Non aesthetic and difficult to remove, swimmers' calculus is common amongst swimmers who train intensively.

Spokesmen of the Academy of General Dentistry, USA, claim that athlete swimmers who swim more than 6 hours a week risk swimmers' calculus. It is a hard brown, organic deposit, often adhered to the incisivo-canin block (Collins and Edington 2012).

Furthering such claims, a study by Suszczewicz et al. (1989) compared 200 school children. Half of them underwent intensive swimming training; the other half had 'normal' swimming lessons. A dark, microgranular tartar was present in 91% of the intensive swimmers, but only in 27% of the control group.

References

American Academy of Periodontology. World workshop in clinical periodontics. 1989

Azodo CC, Osazuwa O (2013) Dental conditions among competitive university athletes in Nigeria. Odontostomatol Trop Tropical Dental J 36:34–42

Collins JF, Edington E (2012) Swimmers risk stained smiles, chipped teeth. Academy of General Dentistry, USA. http://www.knowyourteeth.com/print/printpreview.asp?content=article&abc=S&iid=331&aid=1324. Accessed 25 Jan 2016

Lamendin H (1983) Odontologie et Stomatologie du Sportif. Masson, Paris

Lamendin H (2004) Odontologie du Sport. CdP

Needleman I, Ashley P, Petrie A, Fortune F et al (2013) Oral health and impact on performance of athletes participating in the London 2012 Olympic Games: a cross-sectional study. Br J Sports Med 47:1054–1058

Ozcelik O, Haytac M, Seydaoglu G (2006) The effects of anabolic androgenic steroid abuse on gingival tissues. J Periodontol 77:1104–1109

Socransky S, Haffajee A, Cugini M, Smith C, Kent R (1998) Microbial complexes in subgingival plaque. J Clin Periodontol 25:134–144

Suszczewicz A, Dembowska E, Król J, Siedlecka J (1989) Stomatognathic system assessment with particular reference to tartar in children from swimmer classes in Szczecin. Czas Stomatol 42:311–316

Tavernier JC, Lamendin H (2008) Alvéolyse maxillaires précoces. Chir Dent Fr

Wiebe CB, Putnins EE (2000) The periodontal disease classification system of the American Academy of Periodontology – an update. J Can Dent Assoc 66(11):594–597

Sport, Dental Consequences and Athletic Patients

13

13.1 Introduction

Athletes are equally predisposed to two common inflictions of dental surfaces – dental erosion and dental caries. Both preventable, they provoke acidic demineralisation of the outer enamel layers, continuing to the inner dentin core in more severe cases. Despite these similarities, the two processes are strictly different.

Dental erosion, an irreversible process, belongs to a family of dental lesions of non-carious origin. It is a consequence of lifestyle and its aetiology is multifactorial. Athletes are at risk of erosion of *both* extrinsic and intrinsic causes. Consumption of acid-rich foods and supplements, the presence of gastric acid in the oral cavity and hyposalivation during effort are just a few of the risk factors that increase an athlete's susceptibility.

The formation of dental caries, however, requires the presence of bacteria, notably in the form of a biofilm, sugar and a vulnerable host. It is reversible in its initial stages, unlike dental erosion.

A thorough medical, lifestyle and sporting interview, coupled with a rigorous clinical examination, will guide the practitioner's choice of preventative measures and any necessary symptomatic treatment needed.

13.2 Dental Erosion: A New Epidemic?

Interest in dental erosion is relatively recent, dating from the mid-1990s (Johansson et al. 2012). Dental erosion belongs to a family of dental lesions of non-carious origin which result in the irreversible pathological loss of hard tissue dental surfaces. Their prevalence has been in constant augmentation due to changes in lifestyle habits (El Aidi et al. 2006), and a study by Mahoney and Kipatrick (2003) suggests that up to 43% of adults are currently affected.

S.C. Budd, J.-C. Egea, *Sport and Oral Health*, DOI 10.1007/978-3-319-53423-7_13

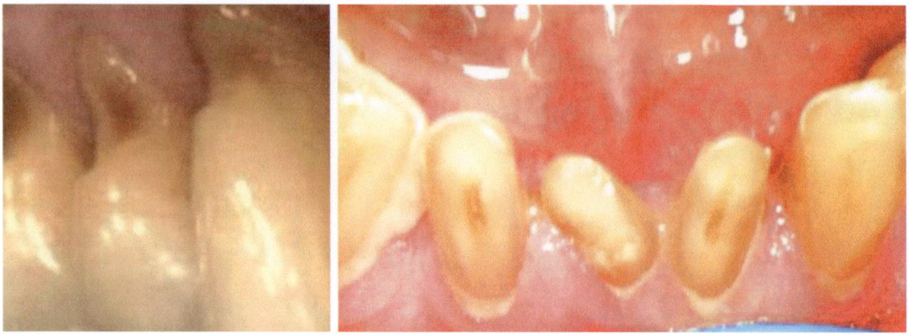

Fig. 13.1 Abrasion and attrition: non-carious lesions

The three main types of non-carious dental lesions are:

1. *Abrasion:* mechanical wear of surfaces, e.g. by overzealous tooth brushing
2. *Attrition*: interaction of dento-dentaire contacts between proximal and occlusal faces
3. *Erosion:* which has been defined as 'the loss of dental hard tissue by a chemical process that does not involve the influence of bacteria' (Pindborg 1970)

The three separate phenomena are interrelated, as Nunn (1996) point out. As the outer enamel layer demineralises, it becomes more susceptible to abrasion and attrition, another vicious circle (Fig. 13.1).

13.2.1 Aetiology of Erosion

The aetiology of erosion is multifarious. It is a consequence of lifestyle. Lussi et al. 2011 distinguish patient-related factors and nutritional factors, influenced by socio-economic status, health, behaviour and time. A global interrelationship exists between individual predisposition and environmental interaction, hence the difficulty to separate one given causal factor.

The pratique of sport and its inherent risks is therefore not a causal element. It is a cofactor that aggravates erosion. Athletes are particularly vulnerable as they are potentially exposed to both intrinsic (internal origin) and extrinsic factors (external origin) which accelerate the process. Figure 13.2 illustrates both general and specific risk factors that facilitate the erosive process. Notice how diet and oral hygiene can help protect against it.

The intrinsic and extrinsic risk factors particularly *relevant to athletes* are identified in Table 13.1. Intrinsic causes include an excess of gastric acid in the oral cavity during sport, gastroesophageal reflux and even bulimia nervosa. Equally, extrinsic causes such as a high consumption of sports drinks or 'healthy' fruit juices/fruit, along with vitamin supplements, can induce erosion. A given athlete may be exposed to one or a combination of these factors (Lussi et al. 2011).

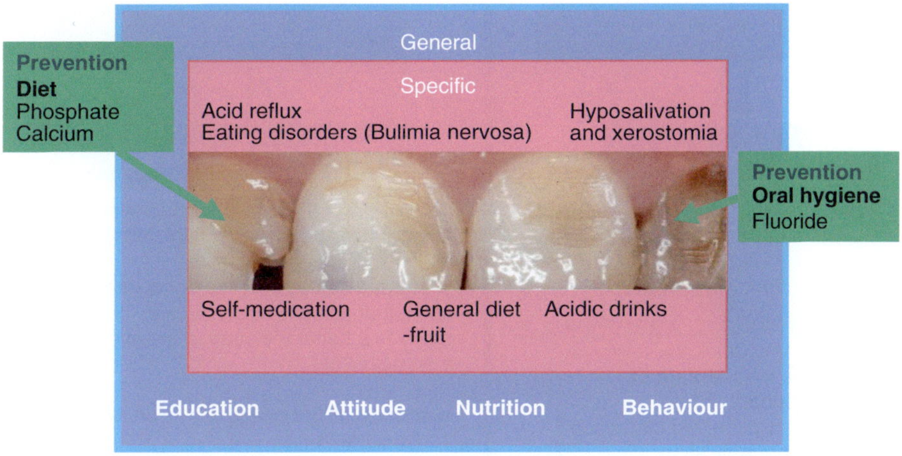

Fig. 13.2 Aetiology of dental erosion

Table 13.1 Extrinsic and intrinsic risk factors of dental erosion relevant to athletes

Extrinsic factors	Intrinsic factors
Acidic drinks	*Gastric acid in the buccal cavity*
Fruit juice, soda, sports drinks	Gastroesophageal reflux (stress)
Acidic food	Anorexia nervosa
Tomatoes, fruit, spicy food	Bulimia nervosa
Environment	*Xerostomia/hyposalivation*
Swimming pool water	Physical exertion
Medication	
Vitamin C, aspirin	

13.2.2 The Specific Vulnerability of Athletes to Erosion

Milosevic et al. (1997) investigated the oral health of 20 elite cyclists. A shocking 85% suffered from dental wear reaching inner dentin layers. Why exactly are athletes so vulnerable? A more detailed diagram, Fig. 13.3, emphasises the negative effects of hyposalivation and the characteristics of popular sports drinks which aggravate this dental epidemic (Lussi et al. 2011) (Centerwall et al. 1986). Swimmers are also at risk when the pH of swimming pool water is below the recommended pH 7–8 (Geurtsen 2000).

13.2.3 The Variable Erosive Power of Sports Drinks

A comparison of well-known sports drinks and their potential erosive capacity has been investigated by several authors. Pinto et al. (2013) found that the average pH of sports drinks was 2.52, more acidic than popular energy drinks. A study by Rees et al. (2005) examined the quantity of tooth enamel removal during a 1 h immersion

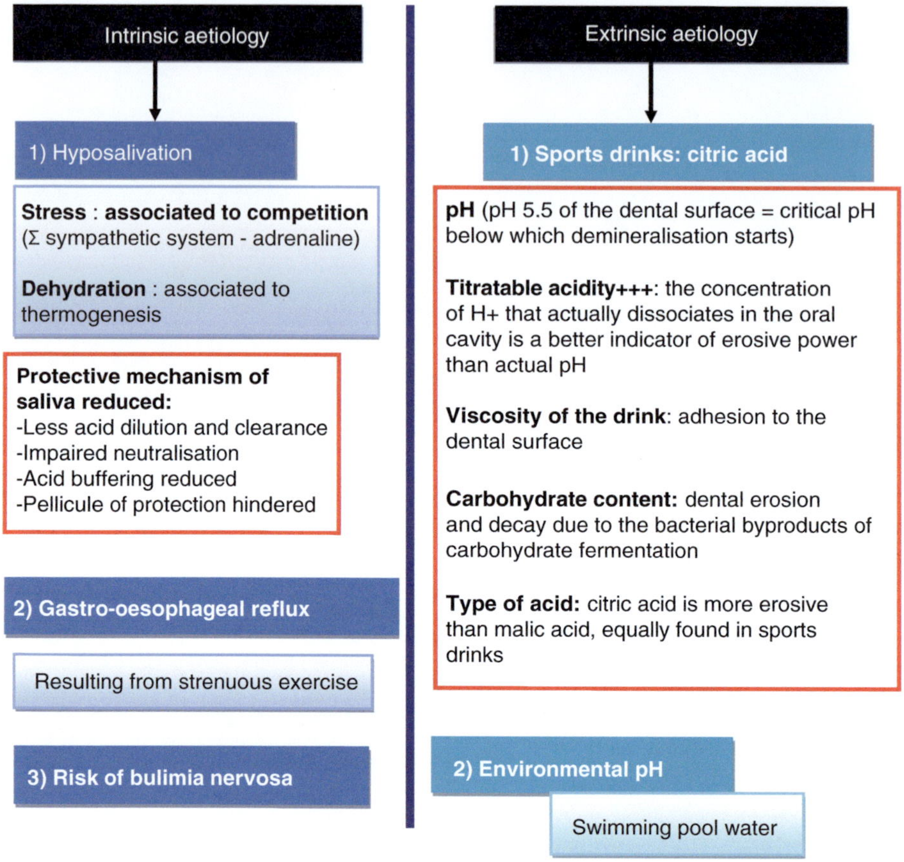

Fig. 13.3 The athlete and dental erosion

in these refreshing supplements. A dissolution of 1.18–5.36 microns of enamel confirmed their erosive capacity.

However, the erosive power of sports drinks is not confined to their pH. It equally depends on their viscosity, carbohydrate content and concentration in protective minerals. Milosevic (1997) compared several well-known sports drinks. A chemico-physical analysis revealed that *all* had an acidic pH value below the critical pH 5.5, hence could facilitate enamel demineralisation. Interestingly, the most acidic sports drink pH-wise was not necessarily the most erosive. This was due to relatively higher calcium and phosphate content. Another important factor is the viscosity of the solution. The 'thicker' the sports drink, the longer it adheres to the dental surface, lowering the pH value of the outermost enamel layer.

13.2.4 The Erosion Process

Erosive demineralisation is initially characterised by the loss of calcium (Ca^{2+}) from the outer enamel layer when the critical pH 5.5 value or below is reached at the

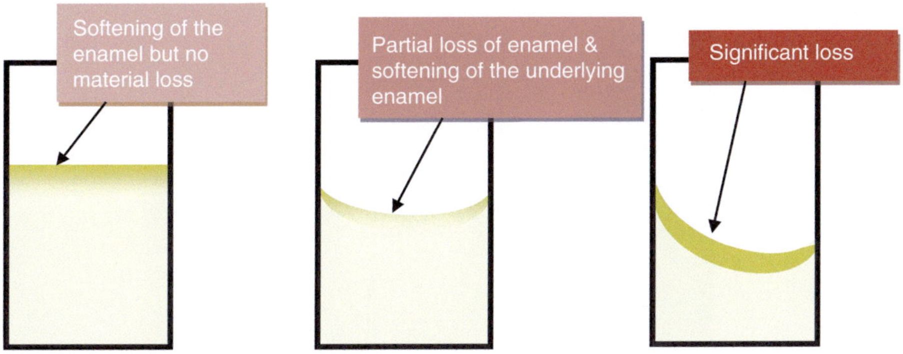

Fig. 13.4 Stages of acidic dissolution of enamel

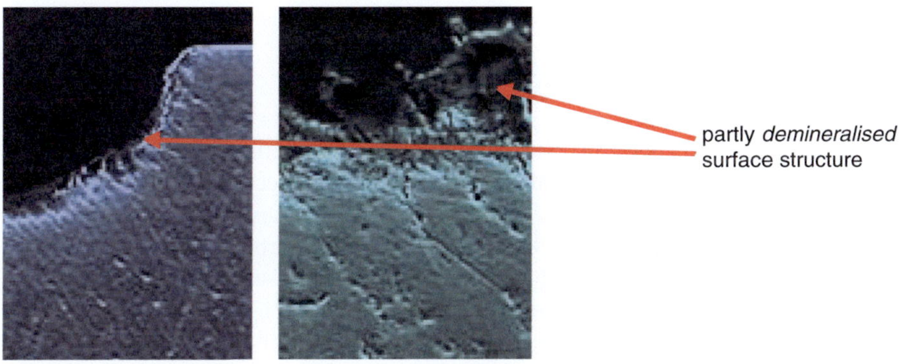

Fig. 13.5 Cross-sectional imagery: demineralisation of enamel

tooth's surface. At first the enamel is softened but there is no material loss. The depth of the affected zone depends on the pH of the given acid and the duration of the acidic attack. As time progresses, the enamel layers are gradually dissolved until, in severe cases, the dentin is reached (Fig. 13.4).

Enamel erosion The different stages of acidic dissolution of enamel:

Figure 13.5 shows electron microscope images of enamel erosion, following immersion in citric acid and treatment for imaging (Lussi et al. 2011):

Dentin erosion Typically, the organic component of dentin is conserved (if adequately hydrated), but the mineralised content decreases with increased and repetitive exposure to acid. Again, the study by Lussi et al. (2011) illustrates this concept. In Fig. 13.6, we clearly see the boundary between the demineralised and mineralised tissue in the cross-sectional imagery. The energy-dispersive X-ray spectra reveal a sharp decrease of minerals in the eroded surface, in particular of the carbon and calcium content.

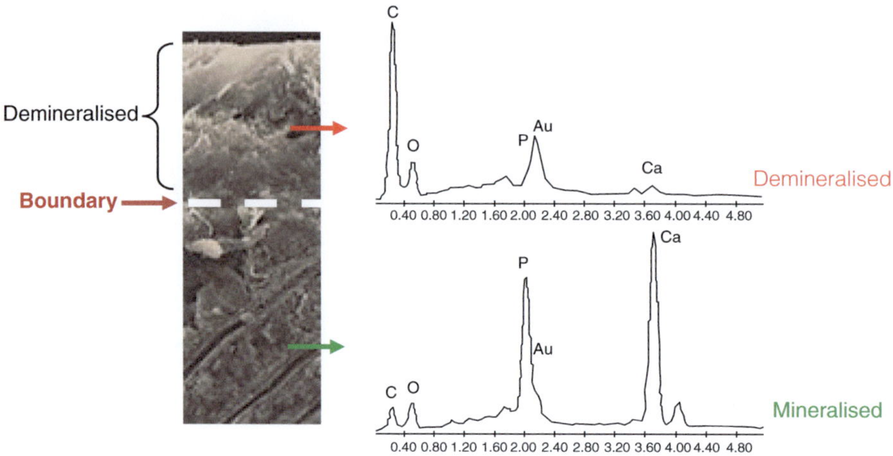

Fig. 13.6 A comparison of mineral content between mineralised and demineralised dental tissue

13.2.5 Diagnosis of Erosion

Early enamel erosion does not cause discoloration or softening of the tooth surface. It is therefore difficult in the initial clinical situation to detect erosion either visually or by tactile examination. In addition, any symptoms in these early stages are often absent or very limited. Pronounced changes in macromorphology occur when the erosive damage is more severe. It is then easier to recognise and the patient is more likely to present clinical symptoms (Johansson et al. 2012).

Thus, for a successful diagnostic and treatment plan of eroded dental surfaces, several parameters must be taken into account: risk factors, aetiology, severity and localisation.

A rigorous anamnesis can indicate the susceptibility of the patient to both extrinsic and intrinsic factors; clinical examination confirms it.

13.2.6 Clinical Examination

13.2.6.1 Characteristics of the Erosive Lesion

According to Lussi and Jaeggi (2008), an eroded dental surface may present the following characteristics: an intact enamel border, a silky appearance, an absence of perikymata on the enamel surface and a characteristically vast spread of erosion in comparison to the depth of loss of material (Fig. 13.7).

13.2.6.2 Severity of the Erosive Lesion: Basic Erosive Wear Examination (BEWE)

Currently, the most internationally recognised classification system of erosion is that of Bartlett et al. (2008) – the basic erosive wear examination (BEWE) system. The oral cavity is divided into six parts (sextants) and all teeth (except wisdom teeth) are examined. Each sextant is given a score of 0–3, based on the most *highly eroded*

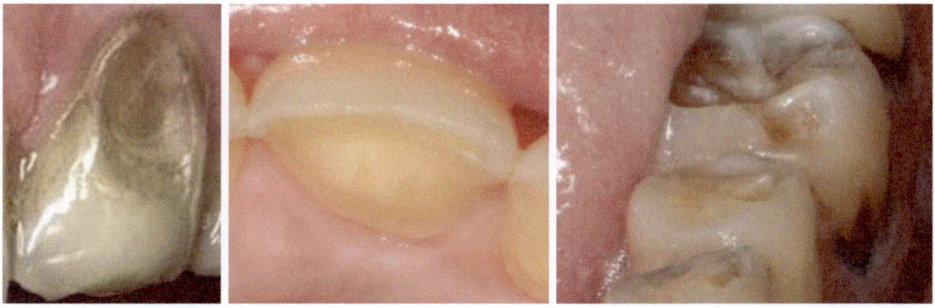

Fig. 13.7 Examples of dental erosion

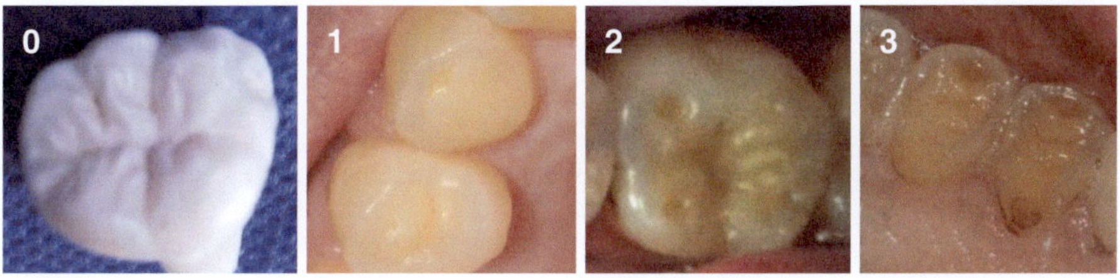

0 : No erosive tooth wear

1: Inital loss of surface texture

2: Distinct defect : loss of hard tissue <50% of the surface area

3: Hard tissue loss > 50%

Fig. 13.8 Examples of the BEWE score 0–4

tooth face in that given sector. An overall, additive score of all six sectors is calculated, giving the *overall risk* for dental erosion. *High risk = equal or greater than 14* (Fig. 13.8).

13.2.6.3 Form and Localisation of Erosive Lesions: Aetiological Differential Diagnostic

The clinical examination of the patient enables the practitioner, in many cases, to diagnose the type of erosion and its aetiology. Preferential locations and forms of tissue loss guide the dentist, enabling a correct diagnosis and eventual therapeutic solution. Figure 13.9 gives an insight into the preferential topography of erosive lesions, according to their origin, whether of an extrinsic or intrinsic source. However, as the erosion process progresses, secondary sites, common to all forms of erosion, may become apparent and therefore confuse the aetiological differential diagnostic (Lussi and Jaeggi 2008).

13.2.7 Complimentary Examinations

In order to achieve an effective therapeutic solution and to monitor progress, it is interesting to use study casts and photographs as a compliment to the clinical examination. Such material also motivates, informs and relieves the patient. They can

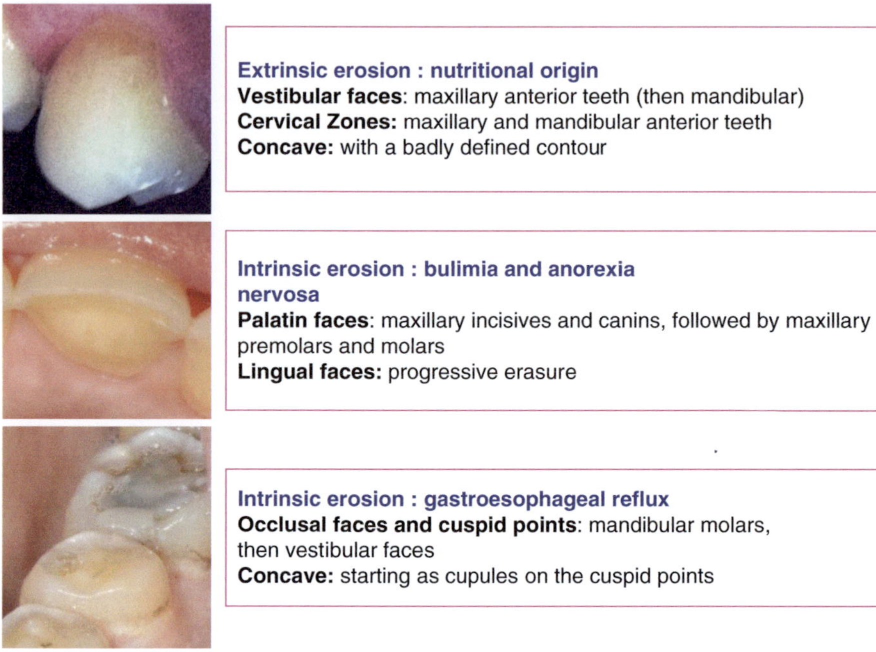

Fig. 13.9 Principal locations and morphology of different erosion types

visualise the current 3D reality of the situation and the interventions required to improve their dental lesions (Milosevic 1997).

13.2.8 Introduction to Therapeutic Solutions of Dental Erosions

The therapeutic solutions of dental erosions depend on the severity, extent and symptoms of the lesions. Possible symptoms include hypersensitivity and aesthetic and occlusal complications. Treatment plans range from prophylactic measures reducing acid exposure to global long-term rehabilitation programmes (Kilpatrick and Mahoney 2004).

13.3 The Prevalence of Dental Caries

According to the US Department of Health and Human Services (1996), 'Of all the infectious diseases affecting humans, dental caries may be the most prevalent'. Worldwide, 60–90% of school children and nearly *100% of adults have dental cavities,* often leading to pain and discomfort (World Health Organization 2016). Unlike dental erosion, a relatively recent concept, interest in dental caries dates back to the nineteenth century, when the newfound sugar availability turned dental caries into a global epidemic (Ismail et al. 2013).

Indeed, Needleman et al. (2013) revealed that 55% of participants at the London Olympics 2012 had irreversible caries – 18% of which said their sporting performance was affected, with even one athlete having to pull out of his event to get treatment. This study therefore suggests that the carious risk of elite athletes is highly significant.

13.3.1 The Carious Process

The carious process, like that of dental erosion, implies the demineralisation of dental hard tissue via exposure to acid. Initial softening of the outer surface enamel starts when the pH of the tooth's surface descends below pH 5.5. However, the mechanism is strictly different between the two phenomena. To initiate dental caries, sugar, bacteria and time are indispensable.

Dental caries may therefore be defined as the localised destruction of susceptible dental hard tissues by *acidic by-products*, lactic acid, from *bacterial* fermentation of dietary carbohydrates. This infectious disease process *is initiated within the bacterial biofilm,* notably *Streptococcus mutans* that covers a tooth surface (Pitts et al. 2007). Fortunately, the presence of the body's natural defence mechanism, saliva, contains minerals such as Ca^{2+} and F^- which facilitate remineralisation in a neutral or alkaline environment.

It is a multifactorial disease, initially reversible in the early stages, and it becomes chronic and irreversible over time if preventative measures are not put into place.

The aetiology of dental caries encompasses numerous elements, ranging from the education and knowledge of the individual, to his genetic makeup, to his daily lifestyle (Pitts et al. 2007). Figure 13.10 represents the risk factors of dental caries but is specifically adapted to athletes.

13.3.2 The Diagnostic of Caries

Given the potential consequences of dental caries, such as intolerable pain, abscesses and generalised infection if untreated, early diagnosis is paramount. Unfortunately, many patients consult the dentist when already in pain that interferes with their everyday activities.

Generally speaking, the patient's motive of consultation and description of pain gives the dentist an initial idea of the severity of the carious process. This is then confirmed by dental examination, vitality tests and complimentary exams.

Initial superficial dental caries are considered reversible, such as a white spot. Unfortunately, once the deeper layers of the enamel are reached, they become irreversible, and symptomatic treatment, as opposed to preventative treatment, is required.

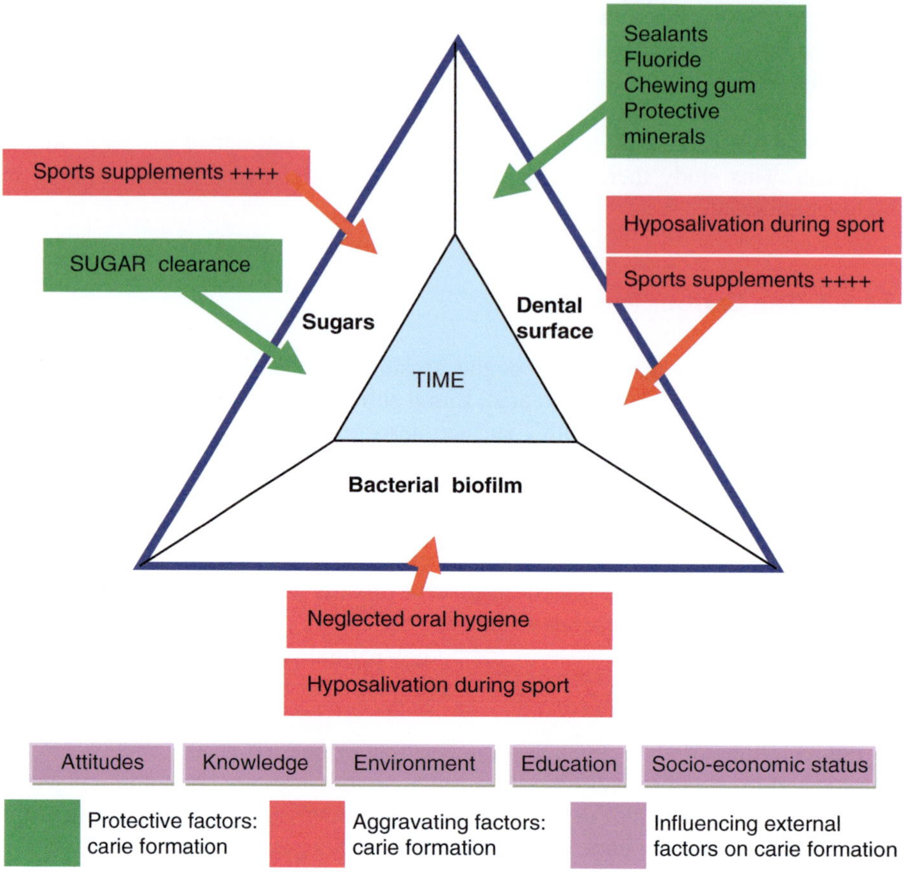

Fig. 13.10 Factors involved in caries development, adapted to athletes

Figure 13.11 shows a schematic evolution of the carious process if left untreated.

The photographs in Fig. 13.12 also illustrate the different stages of dental caries progression. Initial stages are often characterised by the white or brown spots, whereas severe cases commonly include exposure of the pulp chamber.

13.3.3 Introduction to the Treatment of Dental Caries

Dental caries require different levels of intervention depending on their severity and the oral hygiene of the patient. In an ideal scenario, preventative methods would suffice. However, if surgical intervention is required, the least invasive techniques should be employed to help preserve dental tissue whenever possible.

With regard to dental caries and erosions, prerequisite loss of hard dental tissue forms a vicious circle – further dental caries or erosions are more likely. This is particularly true for athletes suffering from anorexia or bulimia nervosa (Colon 2011).

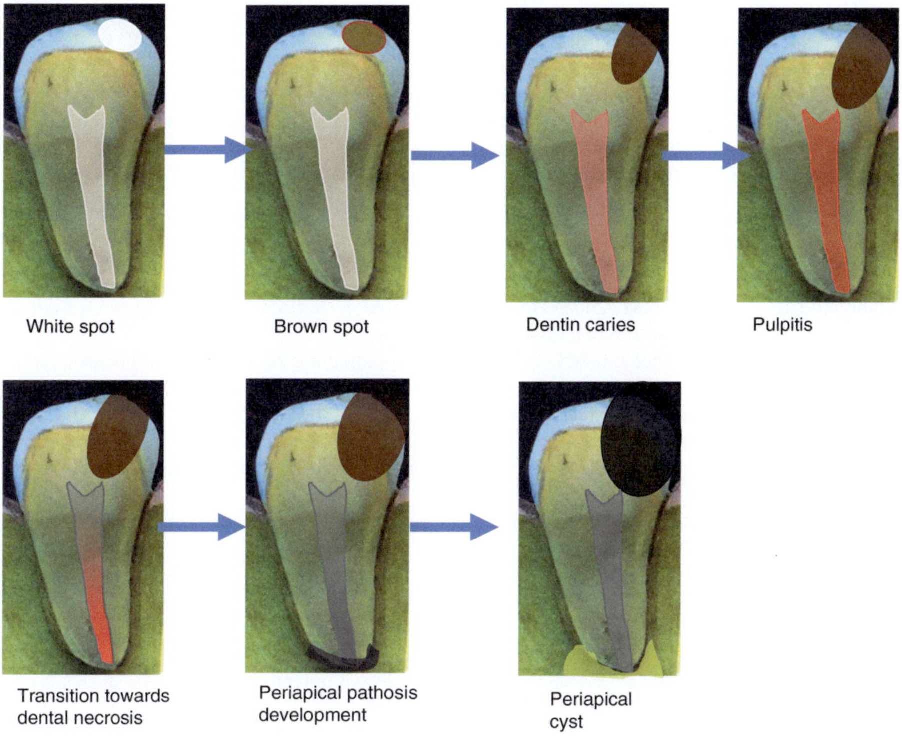

Fig. 13.11 Schematic evolution of the carious process

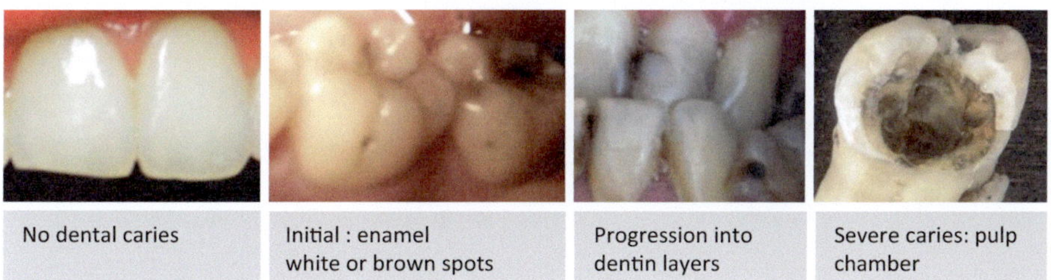

Fig. 13.12 The different stages of dental caries severity

References

Bartlett D, Ganss C, Lussi A (2008) Basic Erosive Wear Examination (BEWE): a new scoring system for scientific and clinical needs. Clin Oral Investig 12(Suppl 1):65–68

Centerwall BS, Armstrong CW, Funkhouser LS, Elzay RP (1986) Erosion of dental enamel among competitive swimmers at a gas-chlorinated swimming pool. Am J Epidemiol 123:641–647

Colon P (2011) Atteintes dentaires consécutives à l'anorexie: quelle attitude préventive? Inf Dent 30:31–33

El Aidi H, Bronkhorst E, Truin G (2006) A longitudinal study of tooth erosion in adolescents. J Dent Res 87:731–735

Geurtsen W (2000) Rapid general dental erosion by gas-chlorinated swimming pool water. Review of the literature and case report. Am J Dent 13(6):291–293
Ismail A, Tellez M, Pitts NB et al (2013) Caries management pathways preserve dental tissues and promote oral health. Community Dent Oral Epidemiol 41:12–40
Johansson AK, Ridwaan O, Gunnar E, Carlsson JA (2012) Dental erosion and its growing importance in clinical practice: from past to present. Int J Dent 2012:632907
Kilpatrick N, Mahoney EK (2004) Dental erosion: part 2. The management of dental erosion. N Z Dent J 100:42–47
Lussi A, Jaeggi T (2008) Erosion: diagnosis and risk factors. Clin Oral Investig 12(Suppl 1):5–13
Lussi A, Schlueter N, Rakhmatullina E, Ganss C (2011) Dental erosion-an overview with emphasis on chemical and histopathological aspects. Caries Res 45(Suppl 1):2–12
Mahoney EK, Kilpatrick NM (2003) Dental erosion: part 1. Aetiology and prevalence of dental erosion. New Zeal Dent J 99(2):33–41
Milosevic A, Kelly MJ, McLean AN (1997) Sports supplement drinks and dental health in competitive swimmers and cyclists. Br Dent J 182:303–308
Milosevic A (1997) Sports drinks hazard to teeth. Br J Sports Med 31:28–30
Needleman I, Ashley P, Petrie A, Fortune F et al (2013) Oral health and impact on performance of athletes participating in the London 2012 Olympic Games: a cross-sectional study. Br J Sports Med 47:1054–1058
Nunn JH (1996) Prevalence of dental erosion and the implications for oral health. Eur J Oral Sci 104(2):156–161
Pindborg JJ (1970) Pathology of dental hard tissues. Scandinavian University Books, Köpenhamn
Pinto SCS, Bandeca MC, Silva N, Cavassim R, Borges A, Sampaio J (2013) Erosive potential of energy drinks on the dentin surface. BMC Res Notes 6:67
Pitts N, Selwitz R, Amid I (2007) Dental Caries. Lancet 369(9555):51–59
Rees J, Loyn T, McAndrew R (2005) The acidic and erosive potential of five sports drinks. Eur J Prosthodont Restor Dent 13(4):186–190
US Department of Health and Human Services (1996) Healthy People 2000: National Health Promotion and Disease Prevention objectives. Full report, with commentary. DHHS Publication no 91-50212. https://www.cdc.gov/mmwr/preview/mmwrhtml/00001788.htm. Accessed 26 Aug 2016
World Health Organisation 2016 Oral Health Fact Sheet Number 318.2012. http://www.who.int/mediacentre/factsheets/fs318/en/. Accessed 16 Jul 2016

The Dry Mouth Syndrome of Athletes 14

14.1 Introduction

The majority of athletes, whatever the sport, complain of xerostomia, also known as 'dry mouth syndrome'. The physiological explanation lies in the decrease or even interruption of saliva secretion in the oral cavity during athletic effort. It is linked to stress, thermogenesis (heat formation) and buccal respiration.

Clinically, the most common dry mouth complaints reported by athletes during physical exertion are thirst, thick stringy saliva, halitosis (bad breath), dry hoarseness of the throat and stomatodynia. Stomatodynia is an irritable, burning or tingling sensation of the tongue or other mucosas of the buccal cavity (Altamimi 2014). Specific oral consequences include cervical caries, periodontal disease and opportunistic infections.

Prevention of lesions associated to dry mouth syndrome includes hydration during effort, dental hygiene and supervision of eating habits and medication taken.

Fortunately, the more severe symptoms associated to modifications of the endobuccal mucosas do not frequently occur in athletes, unless they train intensively or suffer from medical conditions such as Sjögren's syndrome. Optimal treatment of such patients requires multidisciplinary care with medical professionals.

14.2 Oral Consequences

If hyposalivation becomes commonplace, several unfavourable oral repercussions can result. These include periodontal lesions, opportunistic bacterial and fungal infections as well as the development of dental caries and erosion. The cervical band of teeth is particularly vulnerable, as enamel is thin. Oral functions could be perturbed, such as phonation and mastication, and oral defence mechanisms interfered with (Lamendin 2004).

Figure 14.1 summarises the major oral side effects which may be encountered by an athlete exposed to frequent hyposalivation.

S.C. Budd, J.-C. Egea, *Sport and Oral Health*, DOI 10.1007/978-3-319-53423-7_14

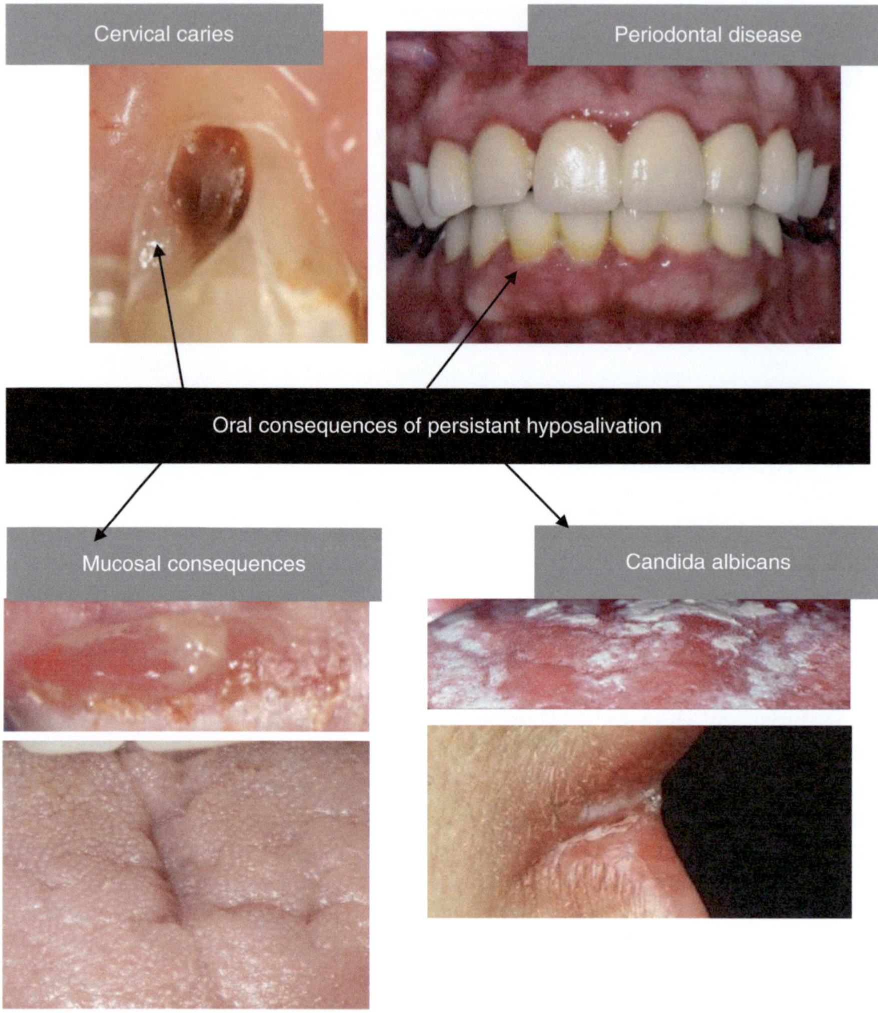

Fig. 14.1 Oral consequences of persistent hyposalivation

- Common mucosal complaints include aphtes and mucosal dryness.
- The main opportunistic infection is due to *Candida albicans*. It takes several forms, including asymptomatic, as a white coating, as a fissured tongue or even erythematous.
- Cervical caries are typical, though all types of caries are possible.
- Gingivitis as a common periodontal consequence (Gonsalez and Sung 2014).

Table 14.1 Simple advice and treatment for dry mouth syndrome in sport

Precaution	Advice and treatment for dry mouth syndrome in sport
Hydration	Sip water frequently before, during and after physical exertion
Alimentation	Avoid acidic, spicy, salty or dried foods Avoid alcohol and caffeinated drinks Usage of sugar-free chewing gum to help stimulate saliva production
Dental hygiene	Regular check-ups Daily brushing and use of dental floss Avoid mouthwashes containing alcohol Mouthwashes and toothpastes containing fluoride
Medications	In severe cases: artificial saliva may be prescribed, though more applicable to patients with salivary gland disorders rather than reversible salivary losses Certain medications used for depression, allergies and high blood pressure may exacerbate hyposalivation
Other	Humidification at night Use of a lip balm during sport: check ingredients such as eucalyptus, menthol, phenol or alcohol which have drying properties *Contact general practitioner or dentist if symptoms persist or deteriorate*

A variety of possible solutions can be suggested to athletes complaining of dry mouth syndrome – either to relieve symptoms or, preferentially, to avoid them in the first place. These range from certain modifications of alimentation to the use of lip balms. Proposals are simple measures to prevent and treat this uncomfortable complaint (Table 14.1).

References

Altamimi MA (2014) Update knowledge of dry mouth- A guideline for dentists. Afr Health Sci 14:736–742

Gonsalez S, Sung H (2014) Oral manifestations and their treatment in Sjögren's syndrome. Oral Dis 20(2):153–161

Lamendin H (2004) Odontologie du Sport. CdP, Rueil-Malmaison

Dental Occlusion and Athletic Performance

15

15.1 Introduction

Many studies support the theory that dental occlusion affects posture, muscular strength and output (Moon and Yong-Keun 2011). Equally, dental interferences increase an athlete's susceptibility to injury of biomechanical origin.

Often it is the excess solicitation of pressure captors, 'proprioceptors' of the oral cavity, that induces a chain of adverse reactions, resulting in postural modification and compensation by the locomotor system. This creates mechanical constraints and imbalances. These biomechanical consequences result in unequal force distribution in the body's lower extremity, the feet, and also affect the symmetry of movement and human dynamics. Certain dental malocclusions, if left untreated, can even affect the development of the upper maxillary and affect the efficacity of cardiovascular oxygenation during effort.

The management of dental occlusion should begin in childhood. Early diagnosis, re-education and interception should accompany facial development during adolescence to limit the need for corrective orthognathic surgery later in life.

To introduce this interesting concept, let us take the example of Carl Lewis. An athletic icon of the 1980s and 1990s, he dominated world sprinting and long jumping. However, in 1985/1986, his performances suffered. During this same period, he underwent orthodontic treatment to correct his dental malocclusion. Was the temporary occlusal perturbation during readdressment of his teeth responsible coincidence or causal factor?

15.2 An Explanation: Occluso-Postural Equilibrium

The body's postural equilibrium is modulated via primary receptors. Otherwise known as sensory proprioceptors, they are found in our eyes, feet and ears. More specifically, the positioning of the head and chest is detected by secondary

S.C. Budd, J.-C. Egea, *Sport and Oral Health*, DOI 10.1007/978-3-319-53423-7_15

receptors. These proprioceptors are found in the masticatory muscles, the desmodontium and the temporomandibular joint (TMJ).

The interference of any of these receptors sparks a chain of adverse reactions, connecting all parts of the body. It is therefore imperative not to categorise the oral sphere as a separate entity of the human body but as part of a finely controlled neuromuscular homeostatic system.

Even a simple dental inference can have adverse effects on the body's posture and equilibrium. This systematisation of consequences can be simply illustrated by certain transversal mandibular movements, known as mandibular laterodeviations.

15.3 Mandibular Laterodeviation and Posture Modification

The proprioceptors in the desmodontium of an interfering tooth inform the central nervous system (CNS) of an excessive force. In response, during closing of the mouth, the mandibule deviates to relieve this pressure felt by the patient. Initially in occlusion only, the inter-incisor point is deviated producing an inversed articulation. If this interference is not corrected, this kinetic abnormality becomes a permanent morphological anomaly, known as mandibular laterognathia. Consequently, certain facial muscles are unequally solicited, resulting in asymmetrical mandibular condyle growth and usage (Lejoyeux 2010). The position of the temporomandibular joint (TMJ) is altered, muscles are unequally contracted, the cervical thoracic chain is therefore imbalanced, and general posture is affected (Fig. 15.1).

Figure 15.2 schematises the mechanism connecting dental occlusion to posture (Perdrix 1997).

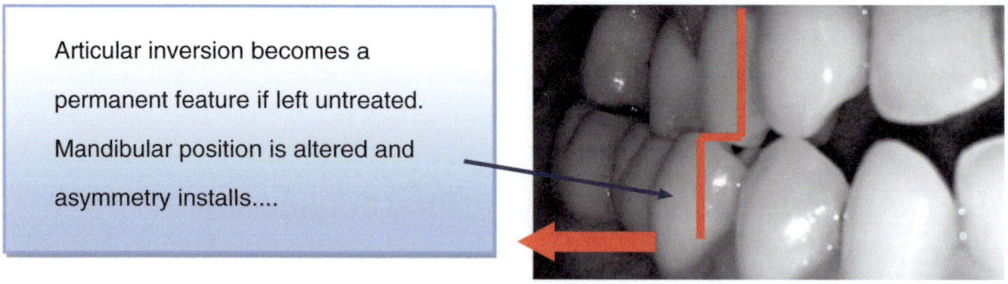

Fig. 15.1 Mandibular laterognathia

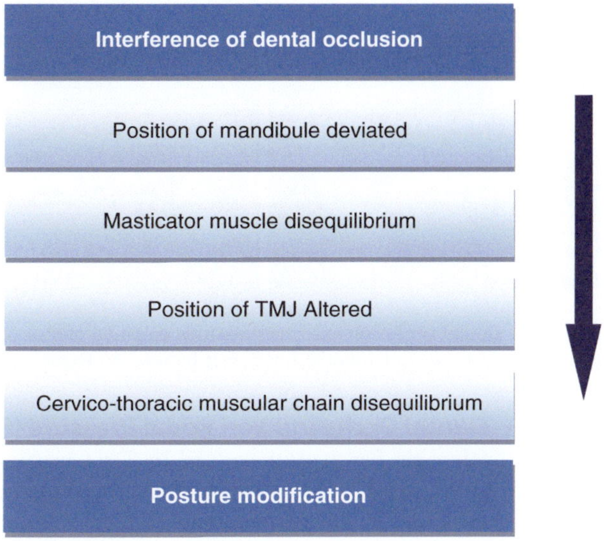

Fig. 15.2 The relationship between occlusal interference and posture

15.4 Connecting Posture Modification and Athletic Performance

How can athletic performance be affected? In response to postural modification, the locomotor system compensates. This induces mechanical constraints of articular, osteo-articular, tendino and muscular origin. The athlete is therefore subject to biomechanical imbalance. This imbalance predisposes the athlete to injury, as mechanical forces are not evenly distributed during impact. In addition, muscular output becomes less efficient, with the non-affected side often compensating and aggravating the situation.

A recent review study by Moon and Yong-Keun (2011) confirms that dental occlusion and the temporomandibular joint can influence the following:

1. The synchronisation of head and jaw muscles with muscles used in body posture
2. Body stability such as body equilibrium (balance), centre of gravity fluctuation and gaze stability
3. *Physical performance and fitness*

15.4.1 Examples of the Biomechanical Consequences of Malocclusion and Altered Posture

Three good examples of how malocclusion can result in impaired athletic performance are the effects on podal pressure, movement and respiration.

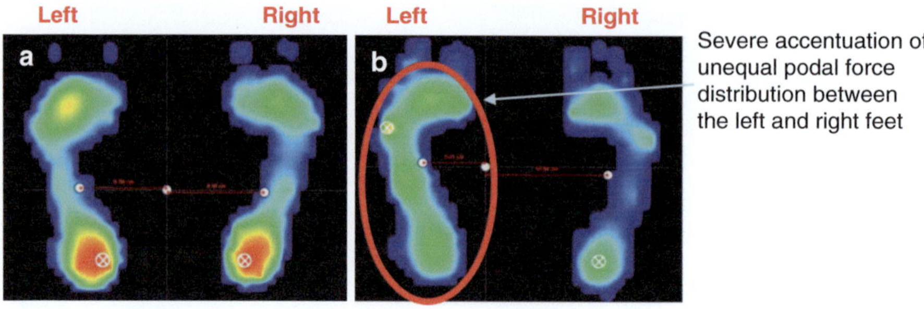

Fig. 15.3 Dental occlusion and repercussions on podal pressure: imagery courtesy of Dr. Valerie Rasigrade 2016. (**a**) Initial podal force distribution. (**b**) Dental scale in place

15.4.1.1 Dental Occlusion and Podal Pressure (Static)

A study by Jerome Farouze, presented by Dr. Christian Pirel (2007), investigated how induced occlusal imbalance or indeed correction influenced the distribution of corporal forces and sports performance of high-level athletes. A dental cotton roll was placed between the maxillary and mandibular premolars of two separate groups, either to balance dental occlusion of the first group or to generate an imbalance in the second. Computerised imaging of podal pressure revealed that in 85% of cases, a direct relationship existed between dental occlusion and podal pressure. He also simply concluded that the group of athletes with balanced occlusion performed better in training and competition than those without. Further podiatric studies confirm these findings. Figure 15.3 shows the distribution of podal forces in an endurance runner. Image A reveals an initial inequality of force distribution, with the athlete applying greater pressure on the left-hand side. Image B shows the effects of a dental cotton roll placed between the premolars sectors 2 and 3 (the left) which created dental malocclusion, 'bad bite' on the right-hand side of the oral cavity (sectors 1 and 4). The inequity of force distribution is severely accentuated. Imagine the same athlete during the propulsive phase of running and the consequences inflicted on the Achilles tendon, the knees and even the hip joints. Injury is inevitable.

15.4.1.2 Dental Occlusion and Movement (Dynamic)

The second influence of dental occlusion on performance is its effect on human dynamics. Maurer et al. (2015) investigated the relationship between different dental occlusion positions, consequent altered mandibular positions and the running stride of 20 athletes. The results confirmed that wearing a corrective dental tray improves the *symmetry of the running pattern*. When specifically adapted to the athlete's dentition, wearing a dental tray may therefore reduce injury risk and improve performance.

A Case Study: Ex-International 5 km and Cross-Country Athlete

An international athlete who represented Morocco in the 1990s, Nadia Ouaziz, supports the results obtained by Maurer et al. in 2015.

She followed a carefully designed, progressive running training programme over 15 years. Otherwise injury free, chronic neck and backache are set in, affecting training and performance. 'It was not so much my performance that suffered, but my recuperation between sessions. I didn't feel rested and constantly suffered from back or neckache'. On arrival in France, an osteopath examined her dental occlusion and diagnosed the source of her problems.

An individualised neuromuscular tray was initially worn both during training sessions and at night. An immediate improvement was noted: 'I had a lot more power in my legs, I stopped swaying from side to side. I felt refreshed and recovered between sessions'. When symptoms subsided, she no longer needed to wear it during training sessions but continued at night (Ouaziz 2015).

15.4.1.3 Respiration and Occlusion

An interesting relationship exists between dental occlusion and respiration during physical exertion. An optimal oxygen uptake is prerequisite for athletic performance, especially during aerobic exercise. An athlete therefore needs a well-developed upper respiratory tract to permit efficient pulmonary ventilation (Boissonet 2011). So how can dental occlusion influence the efficacity of an athlete's respiration during physical effort?

A Case Study: An Ex-International Cross-Country Skier

The following photos are of a silver medallist in the World Masters Cross Country Skiing Championships, Russia, 2005 (Fig. 15.4). The patient currently complains of permanent fatigue and insomnia, an inability to articulate phrases correctly and chronic colds and allergies.

An extra-oral clinical examination revealed a flat profile, long facial type, lip incontinence and flat cheekbones. The intra-oral examination revealed an anterior open bite, a low positioning of the tongue and an underdeveloped transversal component of the upper maxillary part, *associated to buccal ventilation.* A functional examination confirmed pathological oral breathing, as opposed to physiological nasal respiration.

15.4.1.4 Correction of Transversal Growth and Respiration

To rectify pathological buccal respiration, it is the transversal element of facial growth that needs to be addressed. The earlier the interception, the easier the facilitation of

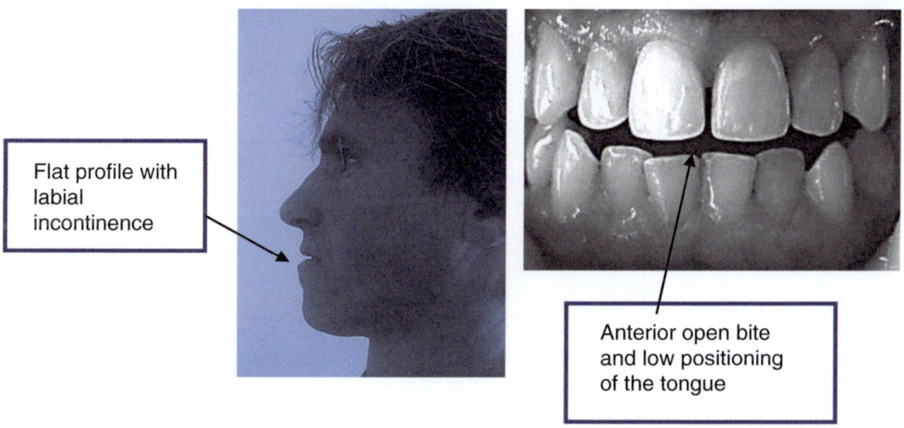

Fig. 15.4 Hyperdivergent profile and anterior open bite in a cross-country skier

correction. Interceptive expansive techniques, such as palatal expanders, are commonly used during adolescence to rectify maxillary anomalies, and are often associated to rehabilitation of the tongue with physiotherapy. Physiological expansion of the upper maxillary enables optimal oxygenation of the cardiovascular system, particularly important in endurance sports that rely primarily on aerobic metabolism.

Equally, overcoming maxillary deficiencies prevents prejudicial repercussions on dental occlusion, notably the development of dental interferences and an inversed articulation, which offset a chain of destabilising reactions, affecting the athlete's posture and locomotor system.

15.4.2 General Principles of Orthodontic Treatment for Athletes

Correction of the transversal component of facial maxillary development forms part of a myriad of orthodontic treatments. The objective is to restore a functional occlusion, a ventilation and a harmonious development of the face. Ideally, molar and canine positioning should conform to Class I of angle. Figure 15.5 presents a patient with Class II, characterised by a pronounced overjet and overbite. In sport, this morphology can predispose an athlete to dental trauma. A well-adapted orthodontic treatment plan can give excellent results.

In cases where the upper and lower maxillary jaw bones are severely misaligned, corrective jaw surgery, known as orthognathic surgery, is a viable option for adults. Figure 15.6 shows the before and after scenarios of a patient with a receding lower jaw. During surgery, the lower jaw is separated from its base and realigned in a forward position. Orthognathic surgery forms part of an extensive orthodontic treatment plan, which involves braces and retainers before and after the surgical intervention.

Obtention of optimal dental occlusion not only restores elements of oral function, such as speech, mastication and aesthetics. It permits neutralisation of dental proprioceptive receptors and postural impediments, essential to peak athletic performance.

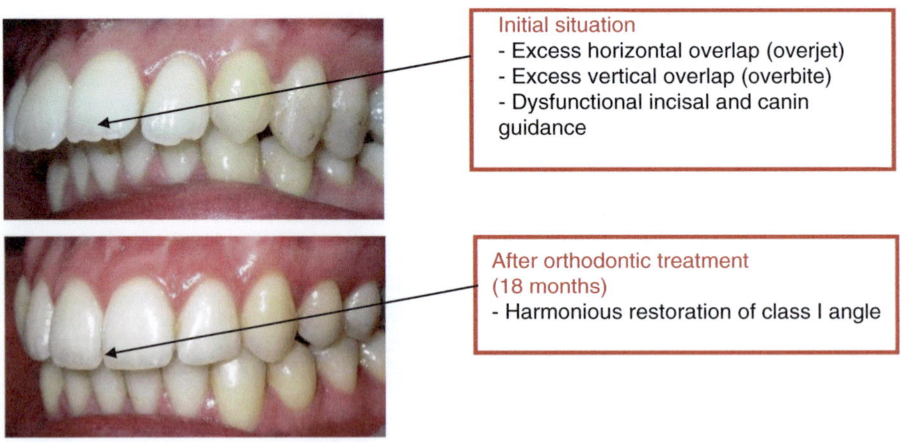

Fig. 15.5 Orthodontics: transformation of Class II angle to Class I

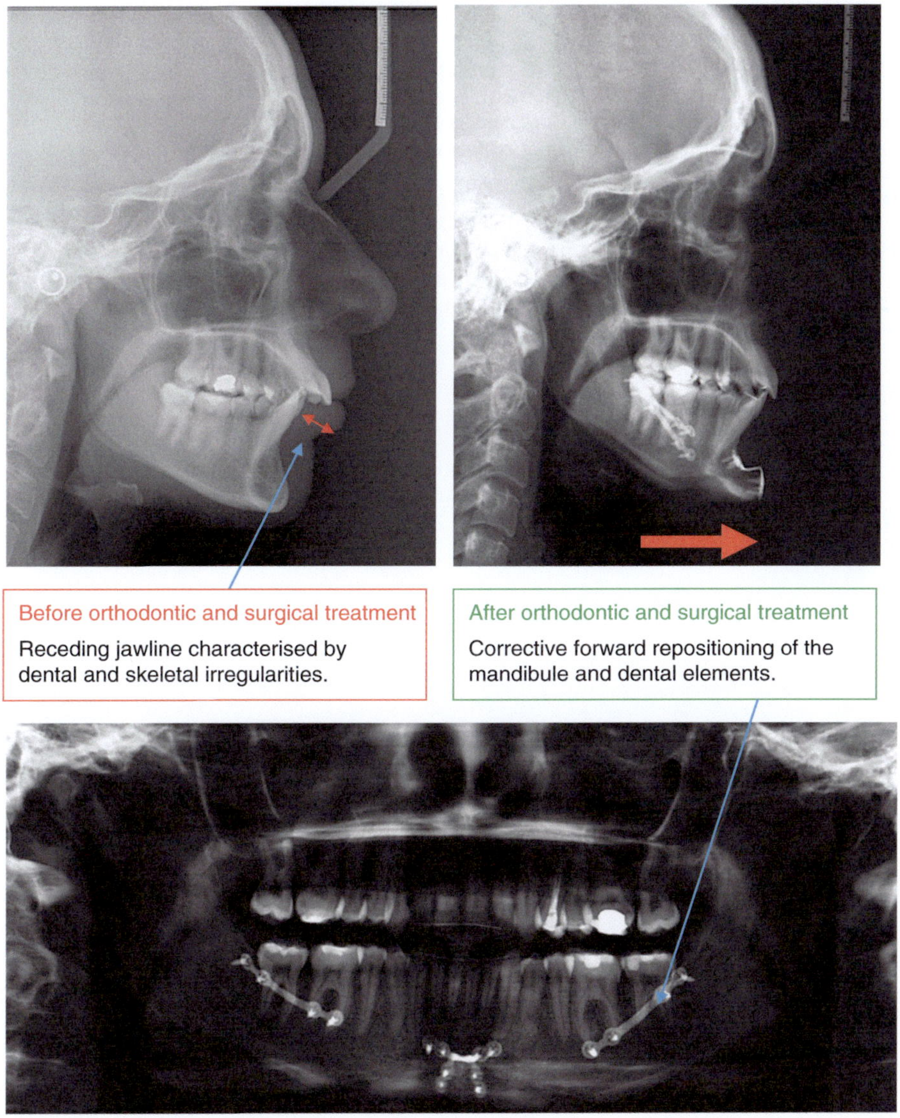

Fig. 15.6 Corrective orthognathic surgery of a receding jawline

References

Boissonet P (2011) Le lien entre l'occlusion, a posture et la respiration. Sport et santé bucco-dentaire. UFSBD. http://www.ufsbd.fr/wp-content/uploads/2014/06/ActesColloqueok_SportSBD_oct2011. Accessed 06 Feb 2016

Lejoyeux E (2010) Lateral functional shift of the mandible and facial asymmetry. Arch de Pédiatrie Organe Officiel de la Sociéte française de pédiatrie 17:985–986

Maurer C, Stief F, Jonas F et al (2015) Influence of the lower jaw position on the running pattern. PLoS One 1(10):e0135712

Moon H-J, Yong-Keun L (2011) The relationship between dental occlusion/temporomandibular joint status and general body health: part 1. Dental occlusion and TMJ status exert an influence on general body health. J Altern Complement Med 17:995–1000

Ouaziz N (2015) The influence of dental occlusion on middle distance running and recovery. An interview. December 10, 2015.

Perdrix G (1997) Sport et occlusion dentaire: influence de l'occlusion dentaire sur les capacités musculaires. Chir Dent Fr 859:34–41

Pirel C (2007) Occlusion Dentaire, Posture et Performances. Table Ronde odonto-stomatologie et sport. Troisieme conference Nationale Médicale Interfédérale. Paris. http://www.franceolympique.com/files/File/actions/sante/documentation/2007/3emeconf-2emetableronde.pdf. Accessed Feb 2016

The Influence of Physical Effort on the Manducator System: Synkinesis

16

16.1 Introduction

The influence of the manducator system on athletic performance is an interesting current issue. Less conspicuous, however, is how physical effort and the locomotor system influence elements of the oral sphere. The concept is inversed. Human dynamics associated to sporting gestures can induce a phenomenon known as synkinesis.

Synkinesis, frequently referenced in syndromes of facial paralysis, becomes apparent when an athlete is pushed to extreme physical limits. A voluntary movement of a specific muscle group can simultaneously induce an involuntary reflex in another set of muscles, elsewhere in the human body. The recruitment of this second group equilibrates the body, relieves muscular tension, increases support and even increases precision of specific gestures. Synkinesis of oral constituents is particularly noticeable during impact – in racquet and ball games, either at the moment of ball contact or indeed with fellow players and, equally, during the latter stages of endurance events when an athlete tires. Movement and repositionment of the lower jaw, tongue and lips are common forms of synkinesis in athletes. This intriguing subject is yet another confirmation of the intricate synergy between various corporal components.

16.2 An Explanation: The Phenomenon of Synkinesis

The term 'synkinesis' suggests that two or more muscle groups, independently innervated, can have either simultaneous or coordinated movements. More precisely, an *involuntary* movement accompanies a *voluntary* movement. The aetiology of synkinesis is not fully understood.

Meyer (1993) defines synkinesis as 'associated movements or involuntary coordinated movements, appearing in a muscle group during voluntary movements or reflexes of another muscle group'.

Currently, scientific literature concentrates on facial and oral synkinesis linked to facial paralysis, as opposed to synkinesis linked to sporting effort. For example, symptoms of Bell's palsy include *involuntary* eye closure during *voluntary* mouth

S.C. Budd, J.-C. Egea, *Sport and Oral Health*, DOI 10.1007/978-3-319-53423-7_16

movement (oral-ocular synkinesis) or inversely ocular-oral synkinesis (Abbas and Pourmomeny 2014) (Nakamura et al. 2003). Equally, the phenomenon of synkinesis is a characteristic of the Marcus Gunn jaw-winking syndrome (Conte et al. 2012) or even Parkinson's disease.

16.3 Connecting Synkinesis, Athletes and Physical Exertion

This concept of synkinesis becomes apparent when the athlete is pushed to his physical extremes. Under the control of the central nervous system, a vast array of muscle groups, not directly involved with specific kinetic muscular contraction of action, are recruited. Involuntary movements of the oral sphere induced by athletic effort facilitate isometric or isotonic voluntary muscular contractions, when the athlete is at maximal effort. In other words, this dissipates muscular effort, relieves muscular strain and readdresses equilibrium. The athlete is therefore ideally positioned for optimal performance relative to his athletic capacity. Various involuntary movements of the oral sphere are *induced by intense athletic effort*. Synkinesis of the mandibule, tongue and lips are common illustrations.

16.3.1 Synkinesis of the Mandibule and Performance (Fig. 16.1)

PROPULSION

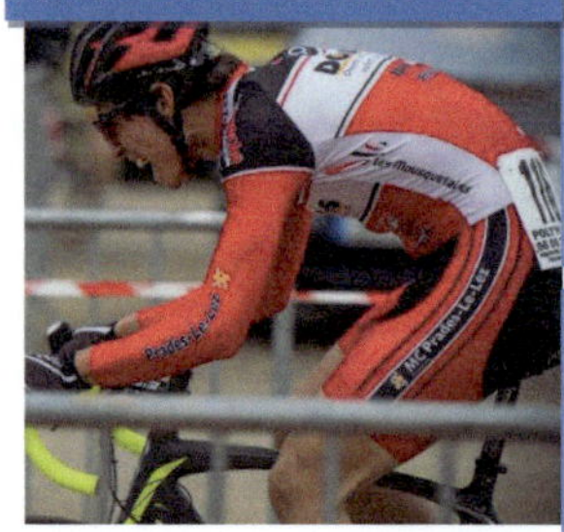

- **Role: forced breathing and optimal oxygenation of muscle contraction**
- Explanation: Elevation of the costo-sternal musculature linked to the hyoid bone increases the diametre of the upper respiratory tract.

- **Role: intimidation of the opponent in competition**
- Explanation: Propulsion of the mandible is a primal instinct of aggression, e.g. rugby.

LATERAL MOVEMENT

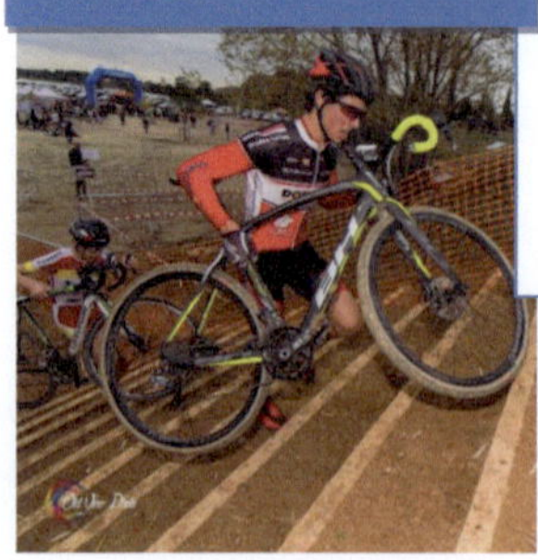

- **Role: equilibrium during suspension movements'**
- Explanation: Reduced tension of cervical musculature readdresses equilibrium e.g. tennis shot, basketball goal, high jump.

Fig. 16.1 Synkinesis of the mandibule

16.3.2 Synkinesis of the Tongue and Performance

The second example of synkinesis involves the highly muscular organ, the tongue. Synkinesis of the tongue is most apparent during endurance events, characterised by an intense and prolonged effort (Fig. 16.2).

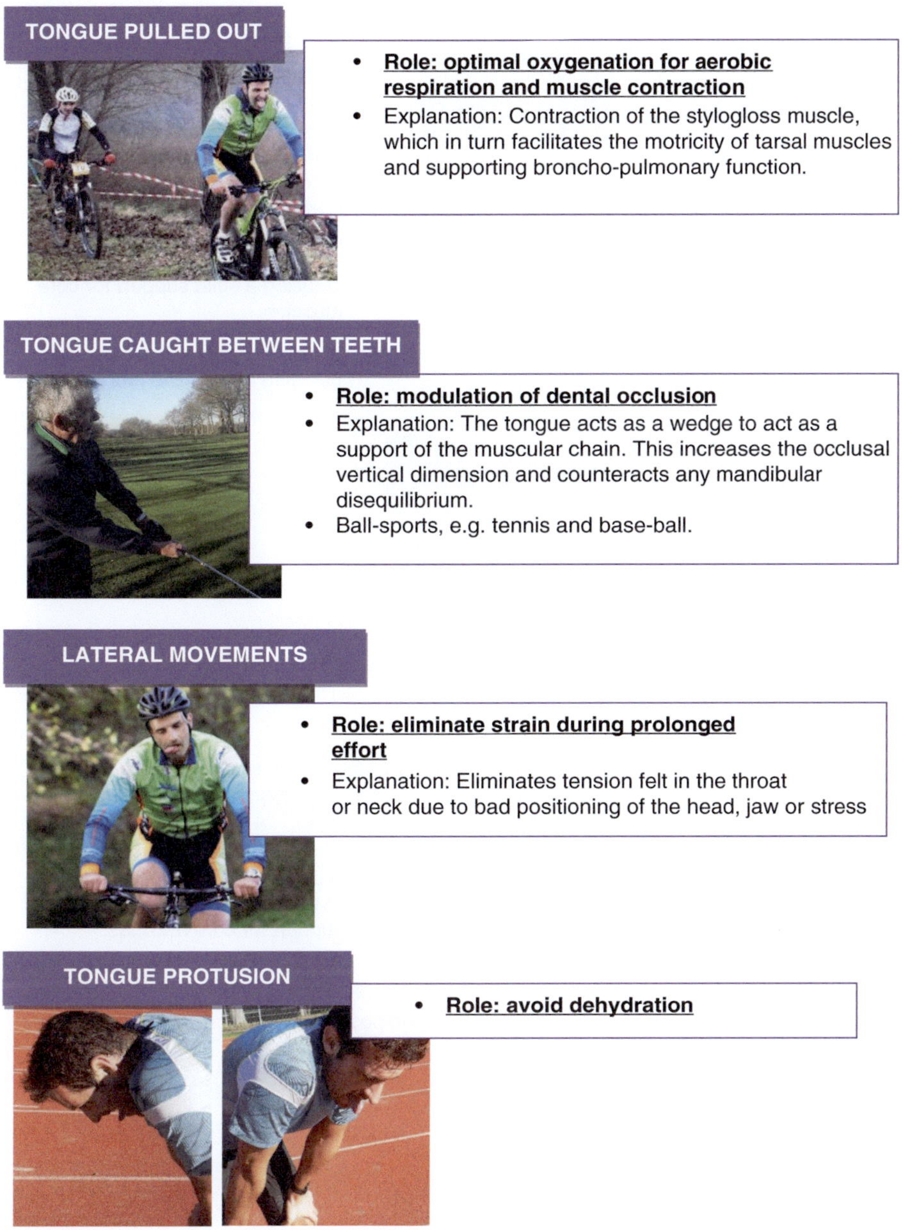

Fig. 16.2 Synkinesis of the tongue

16.3.3 Synkinesis of the Lips and Performance

The final illustration of this interesting concept is synkinesis of the lips. The involuntary movements are more commonly associated to explosive sport or sports requiring high precision (Fig. 16.3).

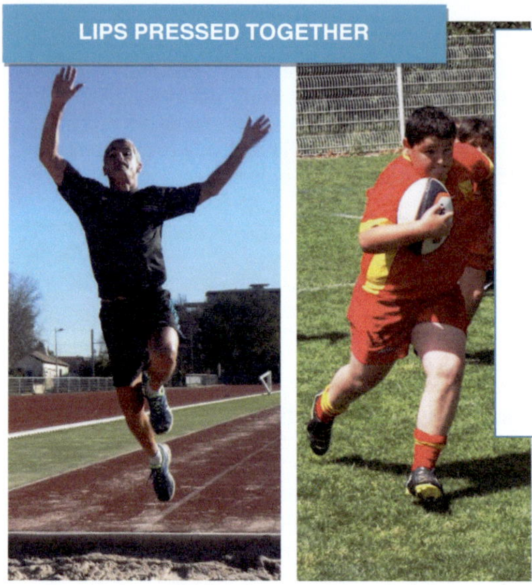

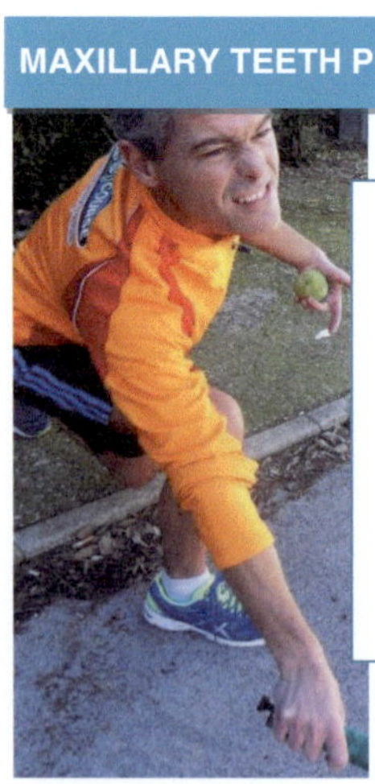

Fig. 16.3 Synkinesis of the lips

References

Abbas A, Pourmomeny AA (2014) Management of synkinesis and asymmetry in facial nerve palsy: a review article. Iran J Otorhinolaryngol 26:251–256

Conte A, Brancati F, Garaci F, Toschi N, Bologna M, Fabbrini G, Falla M et al (2012) Kinematic and diffusion tensor imaging definition of familial Marcus Gunn jaw-winking synkinesis. PLoS One 7(12):517–549

Meyer J (1993) Les syncinésies des élévateurs mandibulaires chez les sportifs. Odontologie et stomatologie du sportif. Masson, Paris, pp 51–56

Nakamura K, Toda N, Sakamaki K et al. (2003) Biofeedback rehabilitation for prevention of synkinesis after facial palsy. Otolaryngology—head and neck surgery: Official Journal of American Academy of Otolaryngology 128(4):539–543

The Spread of Oral Infections and Athletic Performance

17

17.1 Introduction

The relationship between oral infections and their nefast effects elsewhere in the human body has attracted much attention over the years, particularly in periodontal dentistry.

Despite the protective barriers of the oral cavity, micro-organisms can potentially invade mucosal tissues by several mechanisms then reach the circulatory system. Patients with poor hygiene and weakened immune systems are particularly at risk.

This dissemination of oral bacteria into the bloodstream (bacteremia) can damage or cause inappropriate inflammatory immune responses elsewhere in the body known as inflammatory secondary foyers or 'focal infections' (Li et al. 2000). We are therefore faced with two coexisting problems: the spread of both infection and inflammation.

With regard to sport, injuries including Achilles tendinitis, a form of tendinosis, and myalgia have been associated to such pathogen propagation. Deposition of immunocomplexes, toxins and micro-organisms in poorly vascularised zones such as injured Achilles tendons exacerbates existing inflammation, inhibiting the healing process. Injuries become chronic and longer periods of recuperation are required, affecting an athlete's training and subsequent performances.

17.2 The Link Between Periodontal Disease and Systematic Spread of Oral Infection

Research in periodontal dentistry has revealed several links between periodontal lesions and the respiratory, endocrinal and cardiovascular systems. The toxins and bacterial byproducts of periodontal disease have been *associated to* (not causal factors) heart disease (Genco et al. 2001), cerebrovascular disease (non-haemorrhagic) (Wu et al. 2000) and even preterm birth/lower birthweights in newborns via infection of amniotic fluid (Hillier et al. 1991).

Inversely, certain illnesses can induce periodontal disease. For example, Löe (1993) describes periodontal disease as the sixth complication of diabetes.

S.C. Budd, J.-C. Egea, *Sport and Oral Health*, DOI 10.1007/978-3-319-53423-7_17

17.3 The Spread of Oral Bacteria in Dental Practice

It is also commonly accepted that buccal flora crosses the oral barrier during everyday *dental hygiene or interventions*.

Bacteremia results in up to 100% of dental extractions and 70% of root scaling sessions. Even when simply brushing our teeth, bacteremia occurs 40% of the time. In under 1 min, this propagation of bacteria can reach the heart, lungs and other blood capillaries (Kilian 1982).

A pertinent example for the dental surgeon is the well-documented case of endocarditis. Its potentially mortal consequences represent an extreme case of bacterial systemisation. Bacteria of oral origin adhere to the endocardium, causing an inflammatory reaction. Certain invasive dental procedures are prohibited on high-risk patients, hence the need to keep informed on the latest recommendations for dental practice (Glenny et al. 2013).

The dental practitioner must therefore be aware that chronic infections, invasive dental procedures or even routine oral hygiene, such as toothbrushing and flossing, may facilitate the process. Immunocompromised patients are particularly vulnerable, as are patients with ineffective heart valves or vascular diseases (Wu et al. 2000).

17.4 Pathways of Oral Micro-organisms

The oral cavity consists of several barriers to bacterial penetration: a physical barrier (surface epithelia), an electrical barrier and an immunological barrier (antibody-forming cells and the reticuloendothelial system). However, disturbance of the buccal microflora equilibria, often due to poor hygiene and increased dental plaque, can potentialise bacterial propagation and consequent inflammatory responses. But how exactly do micro-organisms and their byproducts escape from the oral cavity? Both bacteria and a susceptible host are required (Page 1998).

It is the anatomical proximity of circulatory systems in the buccal cavity which enables micro-organisms, cytotoxic byproducts and immunocomplexes to enter the bloodstream or lymphatic system with ease (Li et al. 2000). This, in turn, facilitates the development of secondary systematic effects, which include:

1. The *metastatic spread of infection* from the oral cavity via *transient bacteremia*
2. *Metastatic injury* to secondary sites from circulating oral microbial toxins: release of poisonous exotoxins which contain cytolytic enzymes
3. *Metastatic inflammation* caused by immunological injury induced by oral micro-organisms (Thoden et al. 1984): immunocomplexes offset various acute and chronic inflammatory reactions at their sites of deposition

Bacteria have several mechanisms by which they invade mucosal tissues. Either through injured or ulcerated tissue or through invasion of the periodontal tissue

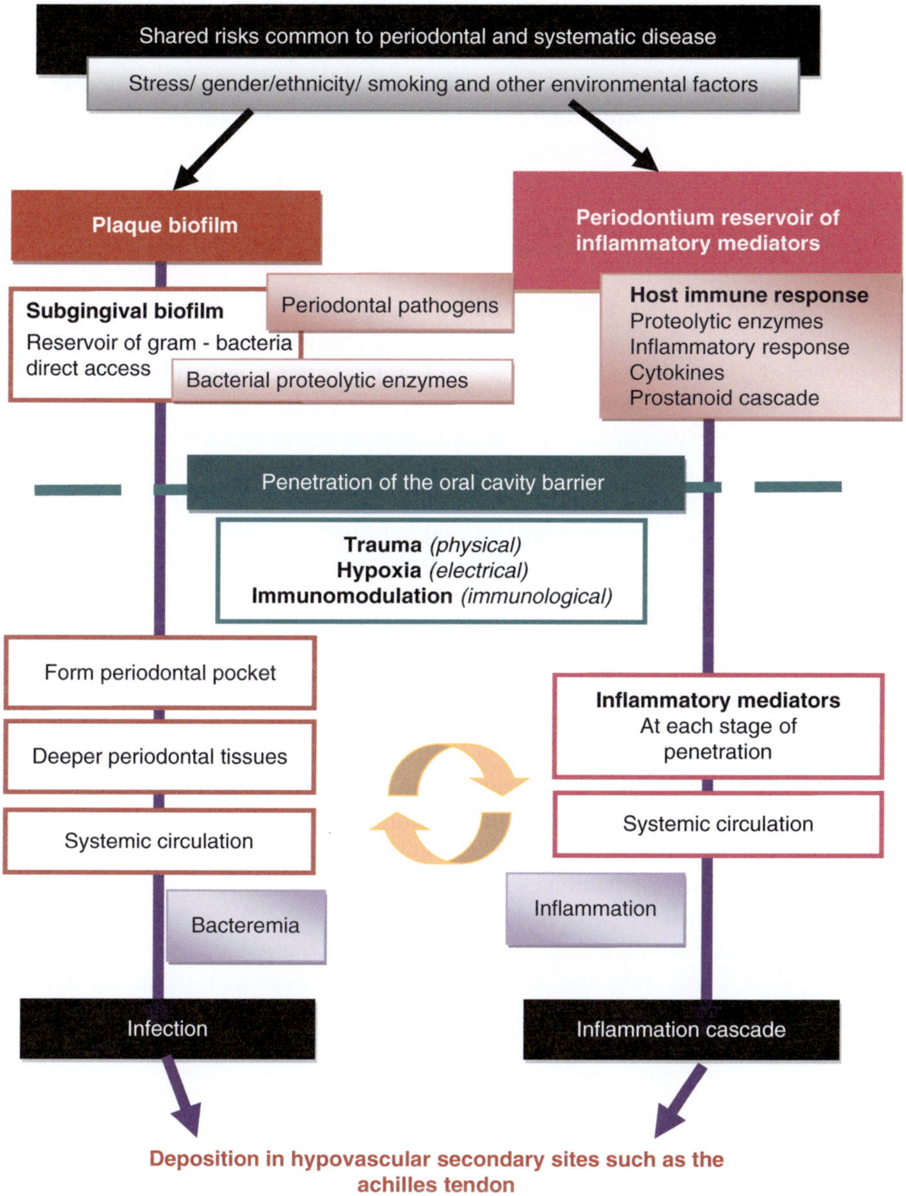

Fig. 17.1 From the oral cavity to secondary inflammatory sites

(Saglie et al. 1988). Figure 17.1 provides a simplified reference to this process. It illustrates the interaction between invading micro-organisms and the consequential host immune response. Tissue destruction is induced at each stage of penetration, and the body's circulatory system is rapidly reached (Li et al. 2000).

17.5 Oral Infections and the Athlete

Specific sporting injuries have been associated to bacterial dissemination in the bloodstream. Prime examples include Achilles tendinitis (tendinosis) and myalgia. It is important to underline that oral infections *do not cause* athletic injury.

17.5.1 The Example of Achilles Tendinitis (Tendinosis)

The aetiology of Achilles tendinosis, for example, is multifactorial. It includes overtraining, unadapted shoes and surfaces and biomechanical imbalances. However, as mentioned, the spread of toxic byproducts of oral infections can cause inflammation at secondary sites. The Achilles tendon is particularly vulnerable as it is notoriously hypovascular zone. Immunocomplexes and other inflammatory elements will therefore have tendency to be deposited around the collagen fibres. This inhibits effective healing of an injured tendon and therefore prolongs inactivity, affecting training and consequent performance. The injury becomes chronic.

Henri Lamendin (2004) postulates two theories to explain this fragility:

1. Firstly, the *allergic theory*: repetitive exposure to germs initially found in oral infections sensitises tendons, ligaments and muscular fibres.
2. Secondly, the *neurovegetative theory*: the autonomic nervous system produces an inflammatory response to bacterial or toxic irritation.

Figure 17.2 photographically captures the connection between primary oral infections and chronic Achilles tendinosis. Oral infection may predispose an athlete to a prolonged injury period.

If an athlete takes precautionary measures as from the initial onset of Achilles tendinosis symptoms, a full recovery can be made within weeks. An athlete, therefore, who suffers from recurring Achilles tendinosis or is subject to a slow healing process, should not rule out the possibility of associated dental problems. Multidisciplinary management of the patient will ensure a correct diagnosis and confirm whether oral infection plays a role.

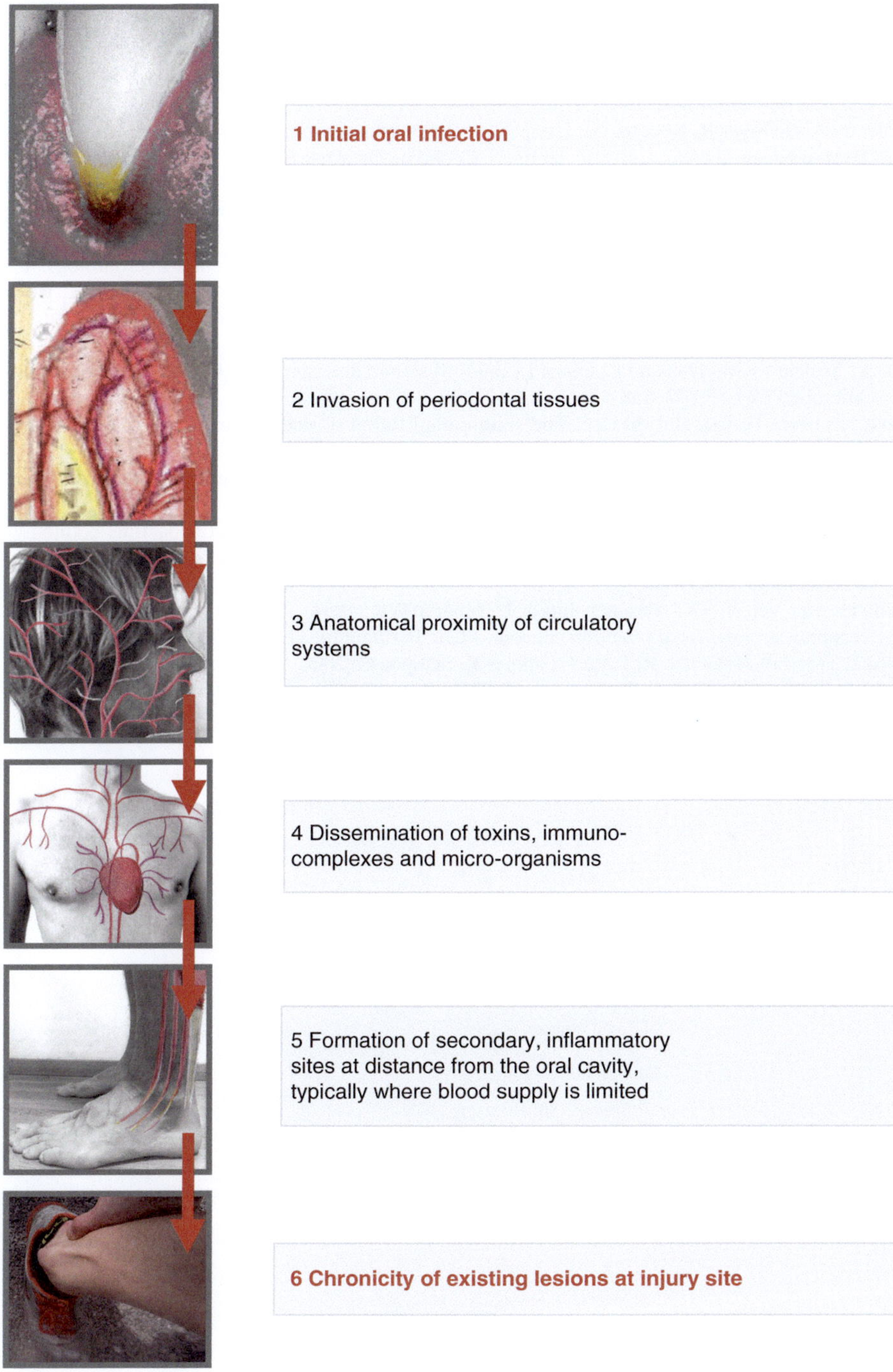

Fig. 17.2 Oral infection and chronicity of Achilles tendinosis

References

Genco RJ, Trevisan M, Wu T, Beck JD (2001) Periodontal disease and risk of coronary heart disease. JAMA 285:40–41

Glenny AM, Oliver R, Roberts GJ, Hooper L, Worthington H (2013) Antibiotics for the prophylaxis of bacterial endocarditis in dentistry. Cochrane Database Syst Rev 10:CD003813

Hillier SL, Krohn MA, Kiviat NB, Watts DH, Eschenbach DA (1991) Microbiologic causes and neonatal outcomes associated with chorioamnion infection. Am J Obstet Gynecol 165:955–961

Kilian M (1982) Systemic disease: manifestations of oral bacteria in Dental microbiology. In: McGhee JR, Michalek SM, Cassell GH (eds) Dental microbiology. Harpers & Row, Philadelphia, pp 832–838

Lamendin H (2004) Odontologie du Sport. CdP, Rueil-Malmaison

Li X, Kolltveit KM, Tronstad L, Olsen I (2000) Systemic diseases caused by oral infection. Clin Microbiol Rev 13:547–558

Löe H (1993) Periodontal disease. The sixth complication of diabetes mellitus. Diabetes Care. 16(1):329–334

Page RC (1998) The pathobiology of periodontal diseases may affect systemic diseases: inversion of a paradigm. Ann Periodontol 3:108–120

Saglie F, Marfany A, Camargo P (1988) Intragingival occurrence of Actinobacillus actinomycetemcomitans and Bacteroides gingivalis in active destructive periodontal lesions. J Periodontol 59:259–265

Thoden van Velzen SK, Abraham-Inpijn L, Moorer WR (1984) Plaque and systemic disease: a reappraisal of the focal infection concept. J Clin Periodontol 11:209–220

Wu T, Trevisan M, Genco R, Dorn J, Falkner K, Sempos C (2000) Periodontal disease and risk of cerebrovascular disease: the first national health and nutrition examination survey and its follow-up study. Arch Intern Med 160:2749–2755

Dental Pain, Life Quality and Athletic Performance

18

18.1 Introduction

Pain is the most common reason for visiting the dental practitioner. Subjective in nature, it can be described as acute or chronic, depending on its duration and intensity. Inflammation, infection and dental traumatology are common causes of pain in the oral cavity, with acute manifestations such as pericoronitis or pulpitis responsible for severe levels of discomfort. Oral pain also varies according to the type of tissue affected. Pain of mucosal origin is typically perceived as a stinging or burning sensation, whereas pain of dental origin is characteristically short, sharp, throbbing or persistent and dull.

With regard to athletic patients, dental pain can adversely affect their performance on very different levels. Intense pain puts an abrupt stop to training and competition. Less obvious is the impact of milder chronic discomfort over a longer-term basis. Subtle interferences arise from diet alteration, sleep interruption, self-medication, loss of confidence and the inability to train at high intensity. Dental pain is one of a multitude of factors that can adversely affect an athlete's quality of life, due to its psychological and physiological implications.

18.2 Dental Pain and Its Evaluation in Dentistry

Pain, as defined by the International Association for the Study of Pain, is 'an unpleasant sensory and emotional experience associated with actual or potential tissue damage or described in terms of such damage'. Pain is not an isolated phenomenon; it is one of the clinical signs of inflammation. It can be described as acute or chronic.

The difference between acute and chronic pain is their duration and often intensity. Acute pain usually lasts hours to days, whilst chronic pain can last months to years and have associated problems of depression and anxiety.

S.C. Budd, J.-C. Egea, *Sport and Oral Health*, DOI 10.1007/978-3-319-53423-7_18

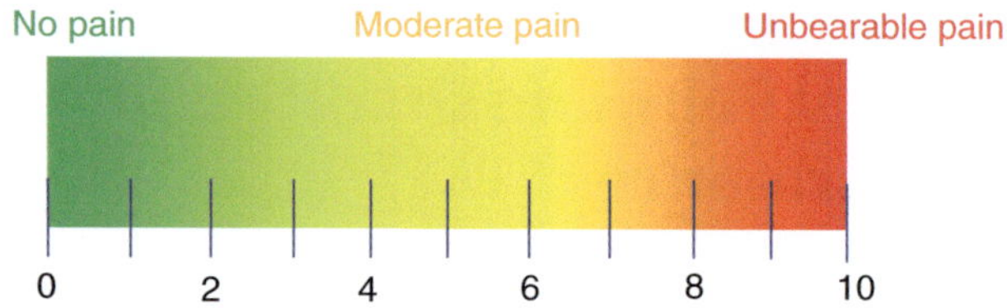

Fig. 18.1 An example of a combined visual and verbal scale used to evaluate a patient's pain

The practitioner's evaluation of pain felt by the patient is an important determinant in the patient's treatment plan. Difficulty lies in the subjective nature of pain. An individual's perception of pain depends on their pain threshold and tolerance, previous experience of pain and emotional state during consultation (Averbuch and Katzper 2000).

The use of visual analogue scales (VASs) or verbal rating scales (VRSs) can help the patient pinpoint the severity of their dental pain (Fig. 18.1). It is also easy for the dentist to under- or overestimate the pain for a given dental lesion (Odai et al. 2015).

18.3 The Causes of Dental Pain

Causes of dental pain are numerous and are of infectious, inflammatory or traumatic origin. The pain felt by the patient may vary from tolerable to excruciating pain, a true dental emergency. Its severity interferes with training and performance to variable degrees. The most common causes of intra-oral pain are recapitulated in Fig. 18.2 (Edens et al. 2016).

Acute pulpitis (1), dental abscesses (2), pericoronitis (3) and facial cellulitis of dental origin are frequently responsible for severe levels of pain amongst patients. As a general rule, perception of pain decreases as chronicity develops (Fig. 18.3)

18.4 Dental Pain and Athletes

Given that most dental pain is preventable by regular check-ups and prophylactic measures, it is a shame that athletes who thrive on peak physical condition often give so little priority to dental care. A study amongst competitive Nigerian athletes by Azodo and Osazuwa (2013) revealed that nearly half of their athletes had experienced toothache; two-thirds reported that dental problems had affected their performance in competition, yet only 40% of them had ever visited a dentist. Equally, a study by Sharma et al. (2012) on the Commonwealth Games held in India revealed that a total of 342 athletes came to the dental clinic during the games. The most frequently required treatment was of a conservative nature: mainly prescriptions to combat pain and infection over the duration of the competition.

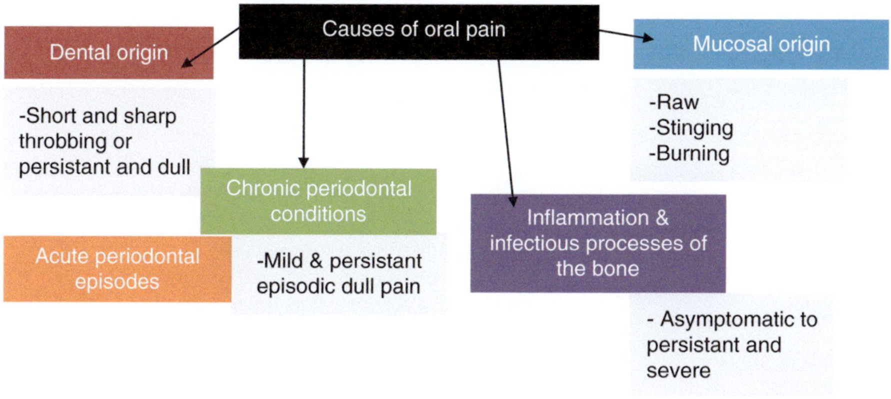

Fig. 18.2 Sources of oral pain

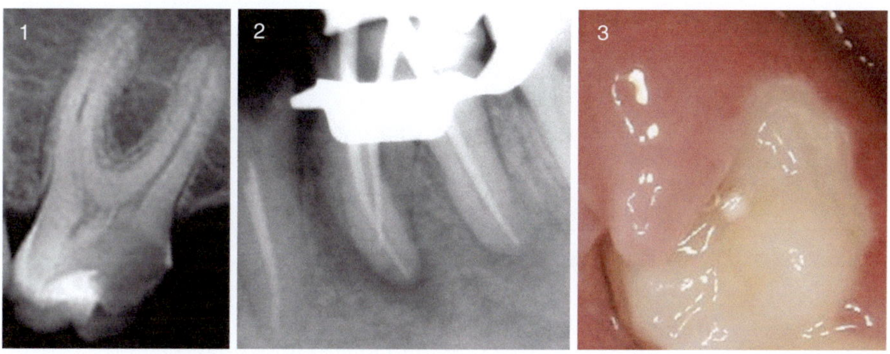

Fig. 18.3 Examples of dental lesions provoking severe pain

In fact, dental pain in athletes has been the subject of many investigations. During the Special Olympics held in 41 sites across the USA in 2001, 13.5% of athletes complained of dental pain – associated to very poor oral health (Reid et al. 2003).

18.5 Dental Pain and Athletic Performance

How exactly is performance hindered by dental pain? Acute pain stops an athlete in his tracks – training or competing becomes impossible and the athlete inevitably seeks help. Less obvious, however, are the insipid, chronic sensitivities, which may not put a stop to activity but adversely affect it. Table 18.1 summarises how an athlete's training and performance may be affected if subject to either acute or chronic dental pain.

Fortunately, negative repercussions on performance are minimised when dental pain is immediately treated. However, as with any other injury, athletes often

Table 18.1 Dental pain and athletic performance

Consequence of dental pain	Implications for training and competing
Alteration of diet	Limitation of required nutrients Morale
Sleep interruption	Mental and physical fatigue Ineffective recuperation between sessions Modulation of immune system over a long period of time Enthusiasm drop Inability to perform at high intensity
Self-medication to relieve symptoms	Risk of secondary effects of anti-inflammatories and antalgics if without medical supervision Implications of doping (e.g. codeine)
Confidence alteration	Drop of concentration levels Unable to deal with the stress of performance
Avoidance of high-intensity training or total stop	Loss of fitness due to lack of training Inability to push the body due to diminished tolerance of pain Interference with training and competition

optimistically think it will 'go away in a few days'. The inevitable development of severe symptoms will then impinge on training and performance on a longer-term basis.

18.6 Notion of Life Quality and Athletes

Dental pain, of chronic or acute origin, is one of several factors that can undermine an athlete's quality of life. The World Health Organization (1997) defines 'quality of life' as an 'individual's perception of their position in life in the context of the culture and value systems in which they live and in relation to their goals, expectations, standards and concerns'.

It is therefore a complex concept affected by an individual's *physical health*, psychological state, level of independence, social relationships, personal beliefs and their interrelation with the salient features of their environment. But how exactly oral pain or indeed poor oral health affect an athlete's life quality?

18.7 The Notion of Impaired Oral Health, Quality of Life and Athletes

Specific elements of the WHO classification of life quality (1997) can be directly related to defective oral health and in particular with regard to the needs of athletes. Table 18.2 focuses upon pertinent areas of quality of life that may be compensated by a complication of oral health.

The relationship between impaired oral health and life quality of athletes has been recently documented by several studies, notably during the 2012 London Olympics.

Table 18.2 Life quality, oral health and athletes

Overall quality of life		
Physical health	• Energy and fatigue • Pain and discomfort • Sleep and rest	**Ability to train, recuperate and perform**
Psychological state	• Bodily image and appearance • Self esteem • Thinking, learning, memory and concentration	**Confidence and sports psychology**
Level of independence	• Activities of daily living • Dependance on medicinal substances and aids	**Self-medication**
Environment	• Accessibility and quality of healthcare • Participation in and opportunities for recreation and leisure activities	**Dental services for elite athletes** **Inability to compete and train**

This study by Needleman et al. (2013) evaluated the impact of oral health on quality of life. They concluded that dental caries in particular had a highly statistically significant association with self-reported impacts ('bothered' by oral health, impact of oral health on quality of life or training and performance). Similarly, data from the 1992 Barcelona Games found a negative effect on everyday life in 41% of athletes (Badia et al. 1994).

References

Averbuch M, Katzper M (2000) Baseline pain and response to analgesic medications in the post-surgery dental pain model. J Clin Pharmacol 40:133–137

Azodo CC, Osazuwa O (2013) Dental conditions among competitive university athletes in Nigeria. Odontostomatol Trop Trop Dent J 36:34–42

Badia D, Soler PA, Batchelor A, Sheiham A (1994) The prevalence of oral health problems in participants of the 1992 Olympic Games in Barcelona. Int Dent J 44:44–48

Edens MH, Khaled Y, Napeñas JJ (2016) Intraoral pain disorders. Oral Maxillofac Surg Clin North Am 28:275–288

Needleman I, Ashley P, Petrie A, Fortune F et al (2013) Oral health and impact on performance of athletes participating in the London 2012 Olympic Games: a cross-sectional study. Br J Sports Med 47:1054–1058

Odai ED, Ehizele AO, Enabulele JE (2015) Assessment of pain among a group of Nigerian dental patients. BMC Res Notes 8:251

Reid BC, Chenette R, Macek MD (2003) Prevalence and predictors of untreated caries and oral pain among Special Olympic athletes. Spec Care Dentist Off Publ Am Assoc Hosp Dentists Acad Dentist Handicap Am Soc Geriatr Dentist 23:139–142

Sharma R, Verma M, Mehrotra G (2012) Dental treatment at the Commonwealth Games, 23 September to 16 October 2010, Delhi, India. Int Dent J 62:144–147

World Health Organisation WHOQOL (1997) Measuring quality of life. Programme on mental health. Accessed 30 Jan 2016

Part IV

Dental Management and Care of Athletic Patients

A guide to caring for patients involved in sport. General principles and the importance of preventative measures. Guidelines for the symptomatic treatment of common dental problems amongst athletes.

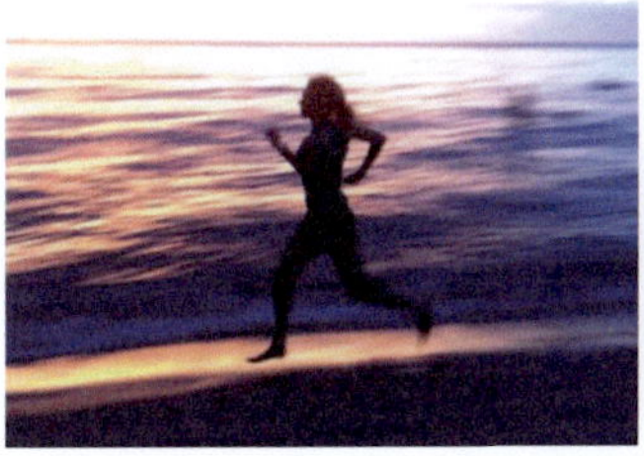
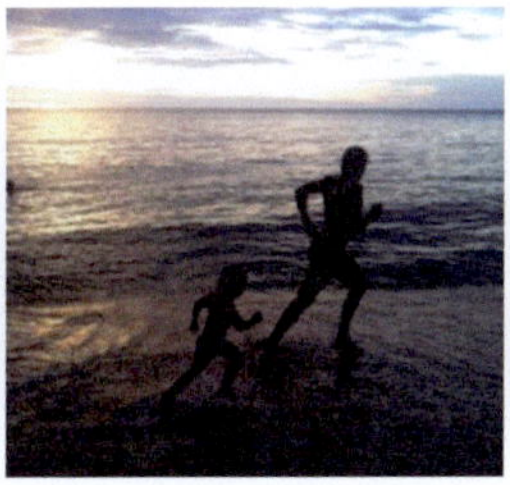
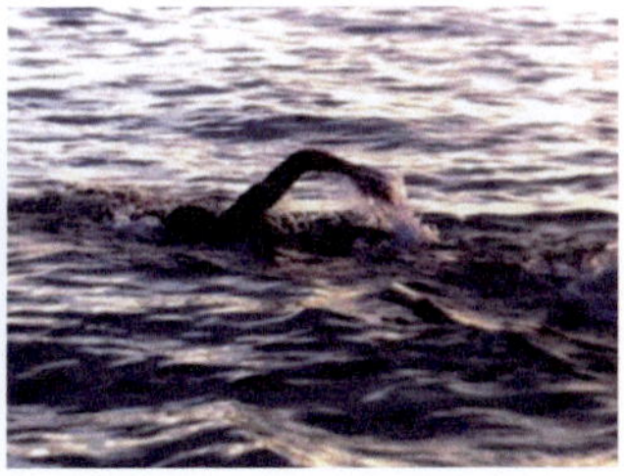

General Principles: Caring for the Athletic Patient in Sports Dentistry

19

19.1 Introduction

Successful management and care of athletic patients requires a symbiosis of several notions. Of utmost importance is the multidisciplinary approach amongst health professionals. Collaboration between a range of actors ensures a correlation of all aspects of an athlete's health.

In dental practice, the practitioner must be attentive as from the first consultation. He must create a reciprocal relation of trust with his patient; he must listen, understand and empathise with their needs.

The clinical examination in sport is explicitly orientated towards evidence of infection and traumatology, dental occlusion and physiological repercussions common in athletes. These include symptoms of dry mouth syndrome or acidic attack of dental tissues. Evaluation of an athlete's individual fragility will permit a precise diagnosis, and a benefit-risk analysis of different therapeutic solutions ensures a well-adapted treatment plan.

The role of the dentist is to monitor and treat all elements of oral health related to a given athlete, to reinforce preventative strategies and to incorporate the athlete's sporting schedule, ambitions and goals.

19.2 The Multidisciplinary Component

A multidisciplinary approach is essential to provide the best care for our athletes. The dentist forms part of a team, which includes medical and paramedical practitioners. These include sports doctors, physiotherapists, osteopaths, podiatrists, dieticians, psychologists and sports coaches.

Athletes strive for physical excellence, but paradoxically oral health standards are often surprisingly low. Whether through lack of education, knowledge, or lack of prioritisation, the role of the dental practitioner has perhaps been neglected, being a less conspicuous actor in athletic performance (Needleman et al. 2015). It is therefore

S.C. Budd, J.-C. Egea, *Sport and Oral Health*, DOI 10.1007/978-3-319-53423-7_19

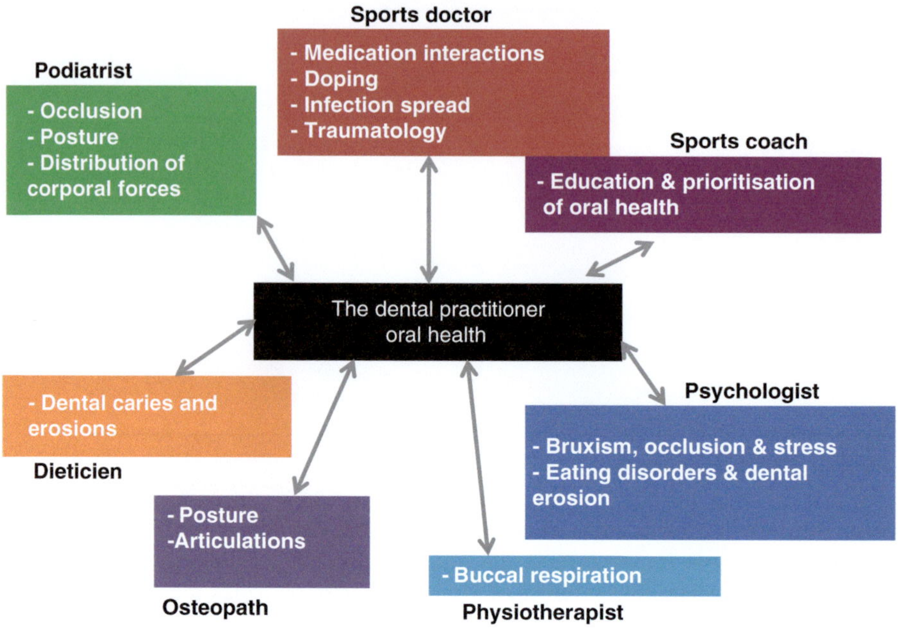

Fig. 19.1 The interrelationship between the dental practitioner and health professionals

imperative that collaboration between different professionals is reinforced, to provide athletic patients with optimal care.

Figure 19.1 emphasises some of the key interrelationships between dentists and other health professionals. The dental practitioner has been centrally placed to highlight the importance of oral health, an element previously overlooked.

19.3 The First Consultation

The aims of the first consultation are to:

1. Form a reciprocal relationship of trust between the practitioner and patient, to listen to the patient and understand his or her reason for consultation.
2. Obtain a maximum of information, whether medical, dental or sporting, to ensure a safe and successful management strategy and ultimate care of the patient.
3. Successfully evaluate individual fragility and predispositions to dental problems, exacerbated by their participation in sport.
4. Start informing and establishing the responsibility of the athlete on all behaviour which could be detrimental to his or her oral health.

It is not just the dentist who must play an active role. In France, for example, the French National Code of Sport imposes that high-level athletes 'must signal all health matters during any medical consultation leading to a prescription' [Article L232–2 du Code du Sport]. They must therefore fully inform the dentist of their medical status.

It is important that the practitioner has ample knowledge and the ability to correlate certain sports medical information to the field of dentistry. A good example is that of Achilles tendinitis. It may be the presence of a chronic oral infection that prevents healing in a rested athlete, a component easily overlooked by doctors and physiotherapists involved.

19.3.1 The Clinical Examination of the Athlete

The purpose of the clinical exam is to observe and palpate hard and soft dental and maxillofacial tissues. The dentist can then detect and diagnose oral health anomalies and form an effective treatment plan to eliminate risk factors and treat existing lesions.

19.3.2 The Extra-oral Exam: Specific to Athletes

1. Palpation of *cervical ganglia*: lymphadenopathy and systemisation of infection
2. Palpation of *masticatory muscles and the temporomandibular joint (TMJ):* muscular contracture and joint anomalies
3. Inspection of *lips:* oral dryness or loss of vertical dimension (labial commissures)
4. *Scars:* evidence of former traumatology

19.3.3 The Intra-oral Exam: Specific to Athletes

1. *Hygiene:* presence of calculus
2. *Periodontal structures:* evidence of inflammation or bacterial entrances
3. *Dental structures:* absent and present teeth, existing restorations, dyschromia, dental caries, erosions, anomalies, malocclusion, malposition, fissures and fractures
4. *Hyposialia:* presence of opportunistic infections, cervical caries and dried and irritated mucosal tissues

19.3.4 Complimentary Examinations to Confirm Clinical Findings

X-ray graphic examinations are indispensable. The maxillofacial panoramic x-rays give an initial global vision of oral health and focus on lesions otherwise invisible in clinical examination. These include the presence of inflammatory or infectious lesions, the positioning of anatomical features and the quality of previous dental

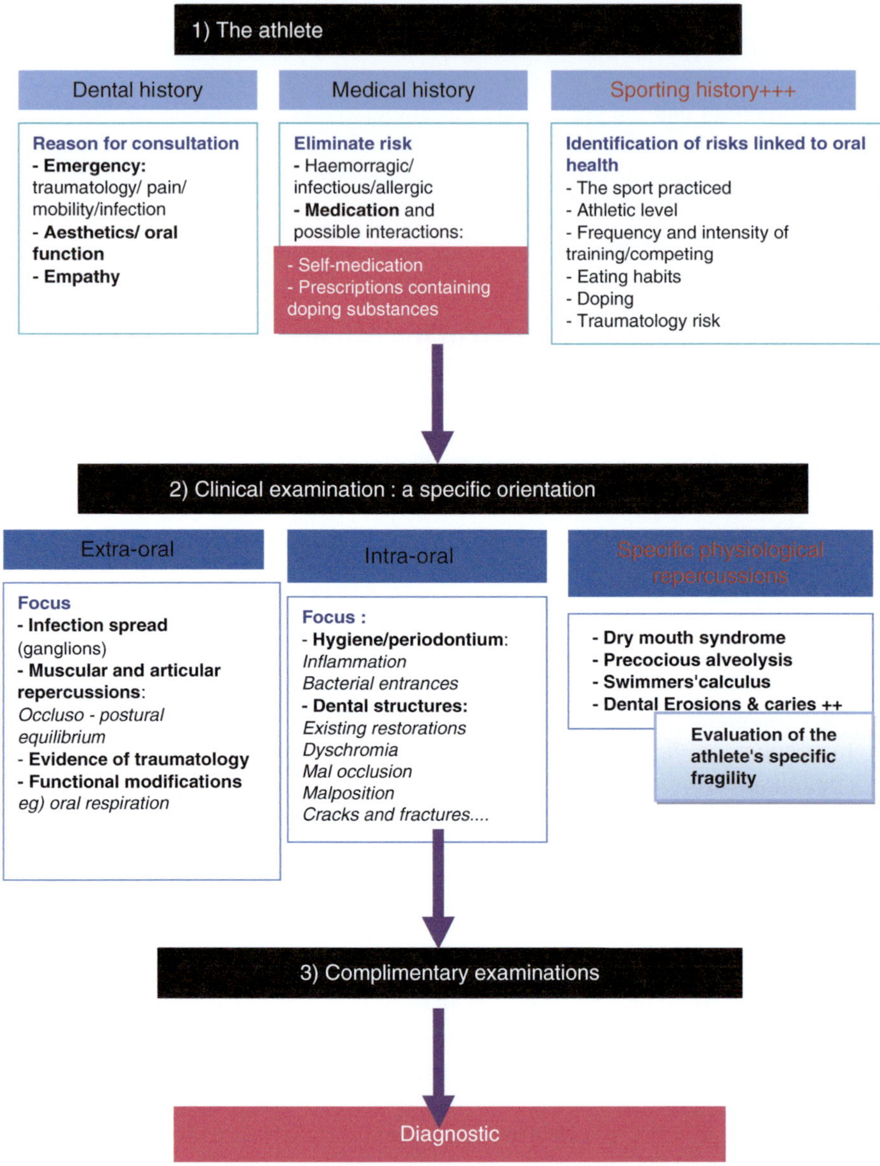

Fig. 19.2 The specific management of athletes in dentistry

treatments. In the presence of dubious lesions, more precise techniques such as 3D scans or retroalveolar x-raygraphy may be used to verify findings.

Figure 19.2 resumes the clinical examination of athletic patients. Compared to the general public, particular attention is given to the intensity of sports practice, possible sports-related risk factors and the search for common dental lesions common to the athletic population.

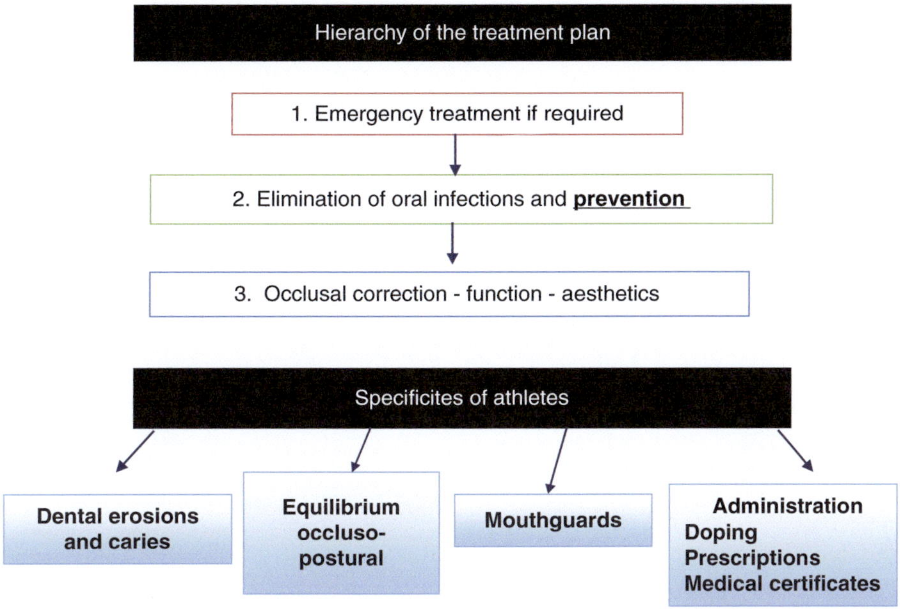

Fig. 19.3 A schematic treatment plan for athletes

19.4 The Treatment Plan

A well-adapted multidisciplinary treatment plan for an athlete is like that of any patient. A certain hierarchy of treatment, responding to the patient's individual needs, enables a successful monitoring and follow-up of dental issues. Initial focus is on the treatment of any emergencies, prevention and the elimination of infection. Then, only in stabilised, healthy oral conditions may specific problems of the athlete be addressed (Fig. 19.3).

Reference

Needleman I, Ashley P, Fine P, Haddad F et al (2015) Oral health and elite sport performance. Br J Sports Med 49:3–6

Dental Practice for Athletic Patients: Principles of Prevention and Symptomatic Therapeutic Solutions

20

20.1 Introduction

As for all dental patients, prevention is the key to sustainable oral health in modern dentistry. Effective prophylactic measures reduce the risk of infection, pain, inflammation and oral parafunctions. Such measures include educating and motivating the patient, liaison with other health professionals and minimally invasive preventative initiatives. Athletes are particularly vulnerable to erosion, caries, specific periodontal diseases, occlusal problems and traumatology. The dental practitioner must therefore inform the patient, evaluate their individual weakness and start implementing prophylactic measures as from the first consultation. A source of error would be to overlook the simple aspects of hygiene such as brushing technique or interdental cleaning. Furthermore, the athletic patient must be educated about the dental biofilm (plaque) and understand the importance of personal oral hygiene.

The specific example of prevention in sports dentistry is the domain of orofacial traumatology. Germectomies of malpositioned wisdom teeth avoid mandibular fractures during impact, and the use of intra-oral protections, commonly known as mouthguards, absorbs shock and shields the oral sphere.

If the athlete requires symptomatic treatment of existing oral lesions, preventative measures are still to be conjointly reinforced. The degree of interception depends upon lesion severity, location and activity. Treatment should abide by the concept of minimalist intervention whenever possible.

20.2 Prevention Management Strategies for Athletic Patients

Figure 20.1 illustrates a prevention management strategy adapted to athletes. The patient must take responsibility for his own oral health, guided by the dental care team. Information is given on dental hygiene and the prevention of pericoronitis, dental caries, erosion and periodontal disease. With regard to sports-related oral health risk factors, modification rather than elimination is sometimes a more

S.C. Budd, J.-C. Egea, *Sport and Oral Health*, DOI 10.1007/978-3-319-53423-7_20

Dental erosion

General

Dietary: reduced frequency of acidic food and beverage intake.

Sports drinks: where feasible, reduced frequency, avoid long retention in the mouth, use straw to drink.

Choose calcium enriched products, water or milk if possible (Carvalho et al. 2015).

Medical history:
- intrinsic aetiology: referral to general practitioner
- extrinsic aetiology: food diary over a specific time-frame eg) 7 days.

Hygiene techniques

Complimentary techniques

Mouthwashes:

-2–3 times a day after brushing for a specific period.

- Anticariogenic, antiseptic, antalgic or anti inflammatory properties.
- Combat periodontal disease, caries and spread of infection.

Dental floss and air abrasion:
- removal of interdental plaque.
- prevention of dental caries of the proximal faces and gingivitis.

Prevention management strategy for athletes
inform - educate - motivate - taking responsibility for oral health

Dental caries

General

-Dietary: reduced frequency and amount of carbohydrate intake. Educate on the harm of frequent snacking of sugar rich supplements.

Focus of drinks of hydration: hypotonic supplements or water.

-Fluoride: toothpaste minimum 1400 ppm

-**WHO:** daily application of topical fluoride, in low doses over a long period is the most effective aget in reducing the prevalence of dental caries.
(Early remineralisation andimproving the chemical structure of enamel reduces the ability of plaque to produce acid).

-Oral hygiene:effective daily dental plaque removal (toothbrushing and interdental cleaning) and engage athlete in prevention at home.

-Regular check-ups: every 6 months if high risk (Featherstone 2000).

Fluorotherapy in dental practice

-Athlete with a high individual risk for caries:

-Fluoride assessment and application of topical fluoride gels or varnishes (eg) Duraphat® or Copalite®).

Sealing of pits and fissures

Unfavourable morphology of pits and the fissures of occlusal faces(Liu et al. 2012).

-Origin of 90% of carious lesions originate from pits and fissures of molars and premolars, both in permanent and temporary dentition (Beauchamp et al. 2008).

-**WHO**: sealants as the reference of primary preventive measures.

Role: prevent the stagnation and proliferation of microorganisms, protecting the underlying healthy tissue from bacterial action (Beslot-Neveu et al. 2012).

Periodontal disease

General

Oral hygiene: behaviour change to achieve effective daily dental plaque removal (toothbrushing and interdental cleaning); use of mouthwashes

Assessment: early detection and treatment

Risk factor reduction: tobacco use cessation

Pericoronitis

General

Oral hygiene: careful plaque removal around impacted third molar

Extraction: extraction of third molar after a maximum of 2 episodes of pericoronitis

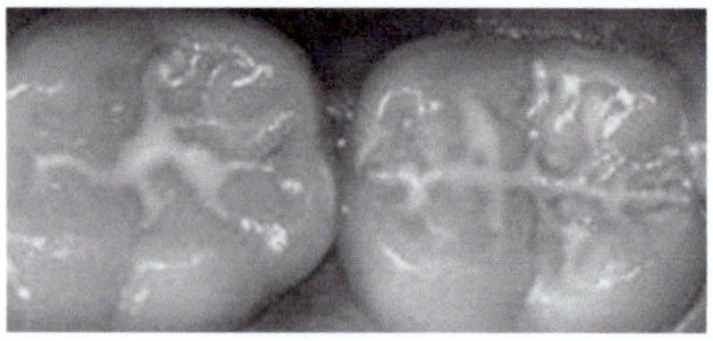

Fig. 20.1 Prevention and risk management of athletes

realistic goal. For example, converting to energy drinks with higher calcium, phosphate or fluoride content as opposed to banning them would be a more practical prophylactic measure against erosion in athletes (Attin et al. 2005).

20.3 A Specific Example of Prevention in Sport: Traumatology

Evidently, prevention is paramount for all dental afflictions, whether the patient practises sport or not. But here, let us consider a specific case of prevention – that of traumatology. Sports, such as American football, rugby and boxing, are particularly at risk. However, participants in endurance sports such as cycling are not immune to accidents.

Two major examples of preventative methods are germectomies and intra-oral protections to reduce the risk of maxillofacial trauma.

20.3.1 Germectomies

Preventative germectomies of wisdom teeth, particularly mandibular wisdom teeth, are typically performed on high-level adolescent athletes. Their indication arises around the age of 14. Panoramic x-ray graphic imagery reveals potential eruption complications due to their positioning or inadequate space. An informed patient may opt for a germectomy as it is a simpler intervention than the removal of fully formed impacted teeth. The significant risk of mandibular fractures associated to unerupted or impacted teeth (Murat et al. 2007) would be avoided (Fig. 20.2), as would displacement of adjacent teeth and painful inflammatory and infectious pericoronitis associated to eruption accidents (Lamendin 2004).

The dentist is therefore responsible for taking regular panoramic x-ray controls to follow up the progression of wisdom teeth calcification. The athlete must be aware of the risks of impacted teeth and be conscious of this preventative solution.

20.3.2 Intra-oral Protections (Mouthguards)

The American Academy of Pediatric Dentistry (2013) insists on the importance of mouthguards for young athletes participating in high- and moderate-risk sports. These pertinent guidelines are for dental practitioners but also for everyone involved in sport. They need not be limited to children but extended to sportsmen and women of all ages. Table 20.1 recapitulates the main recommendations.

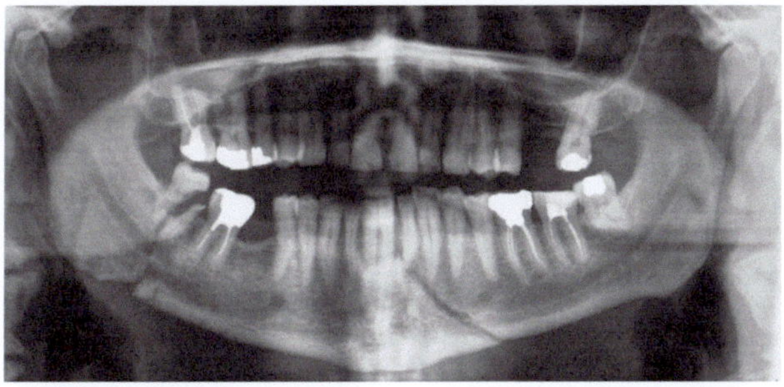

Fig. 20.2 Mandibular fractures in sport

Table 20.1 Measures to promote intra-oral protection amongst athletes

Prevention measure	Policy statement
The dentist and public education	The importance of protective measures such as mouthguards to prevent injury in both sporting events and recreational activities Educate parents and patients on oral trauma prevention
Coaches/administrators	To consult a dentist in preseason practice to obtain the latest information on preventative measures and how to deal with immediate dental trauma, such as avulsed teeth
The dentist and prescription	To evaluate risk and prescribe mouthguards (or referral) for athletes particularly at risk
Promotion of mouthguards	Collaboration with other health professionals, schools, coaches and athletic peers to encourage the use of mouthguards

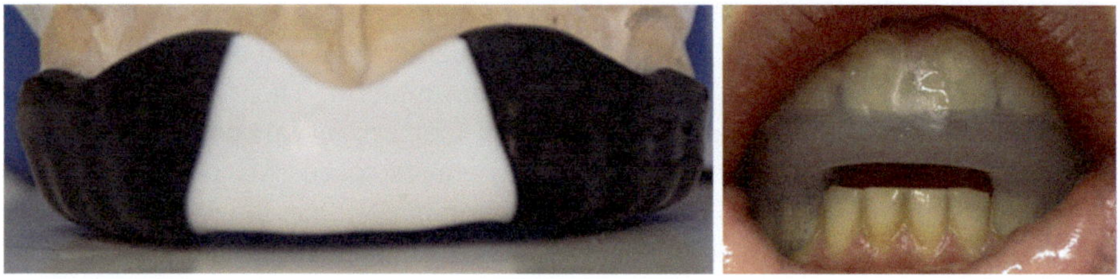

Fig. 20.3 Individualised mouthguards made from dental impressions

The two main roles of intra-oral protections are:

1. To assure functional imperatives such as respiration and phonetics during sporting practice
2. To reduce accidental damage to oral, facial, cerebral and vertebral structures

They protect, isolate and solidarize these anatomical elements, absorbing shock at impact. Currently, there are four available types of mouthguards. Most mouthguards in all of these categories are made from ethylene vinyl acetate (EVA) material (American Society for Testing and Materials 1986). The most effective are individually adapted to the patient and based on initial dental impressions (Fig. 20.3).

The roles of the dental practitioner are:

- To evaluate the type of mouthguard required according to the risk imposed by the chosen sport
- To educate the athlete of the risks of traumatology imposed by his sport and level of participation
- Assure optimal oral health of the athlete before fabrication of an intra-oral protection
- To clinically adapt the mouthguard to the individual: to respect efficient ventilation and assure comfort and function

20.4 Principles of Therapeutic Solutions for Common Hard Tissue Dental Lesions in Athletes: Erosions and Dental Caries

The successful management of hard tissue dental lesions depends upon their severity, the number of lesions and their cause. Optimised treatment planning involves a combination of prevention, protection, interception, temporisation and restoration (Colon and Lussi 2014).

Figure 20.4 schematises the main considerations for athletic patients who present existing lesions. Symptomatic treatment relieves, but an aetiological diagnostic is also primordial to limit further propagation and development of oral problems.

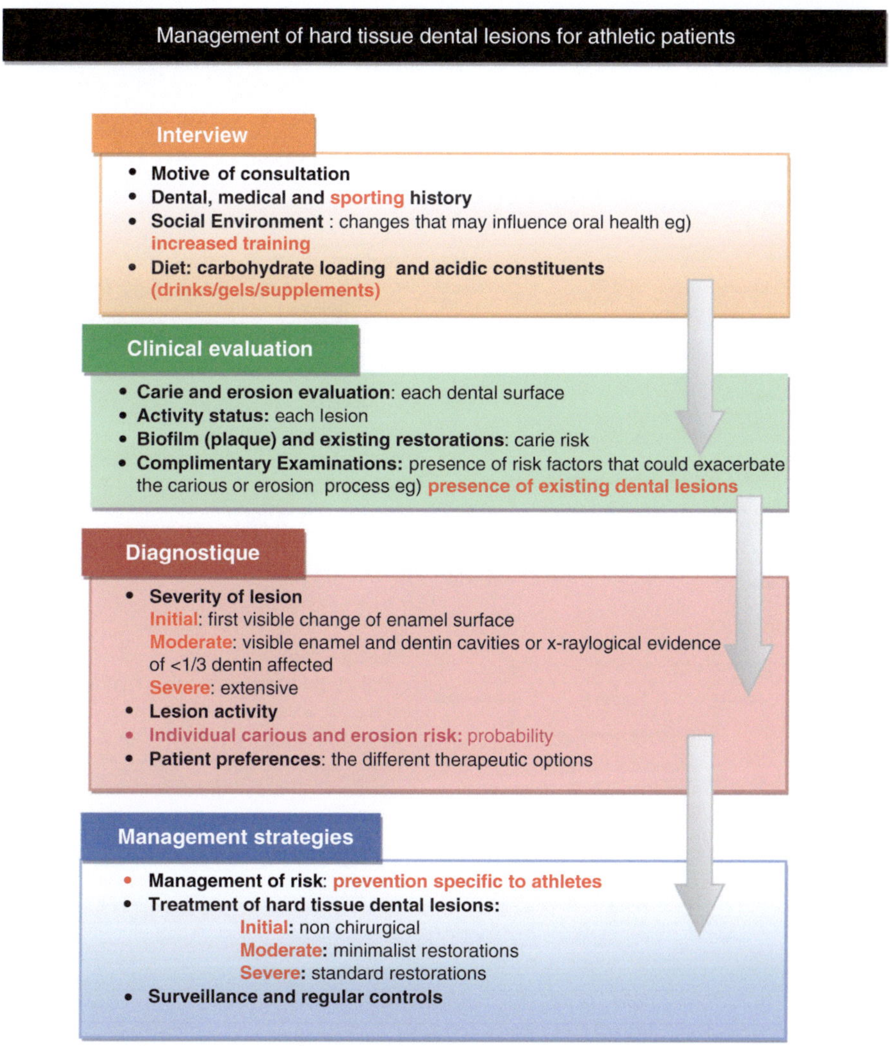

Fig. 20.4 General principles of management of dental caries and erosions in athletes

20.5 Symptomatic Treatment

Restorative management is to reduce or stop progression of more advanced lesions, to alleviate symptoms such as dentin hypersensitivity and to restore aesthetics and function (Carvalho et al. 2015). The aim is to use the least invasive technique possible and to isolate dental surfaces from the aggressive acidic environment. These include direct restorations (composites) and indirect restorations (composite, ceramic and metallic restorations) (Bartlett et al. 2008; Lasfargues and Colon 2010). As severity increases, so does the level of intervention (Fig. 20.5). Symptomatic treatment should be used in conjunction with preventative measures at all times (Ismail et al. 2013).

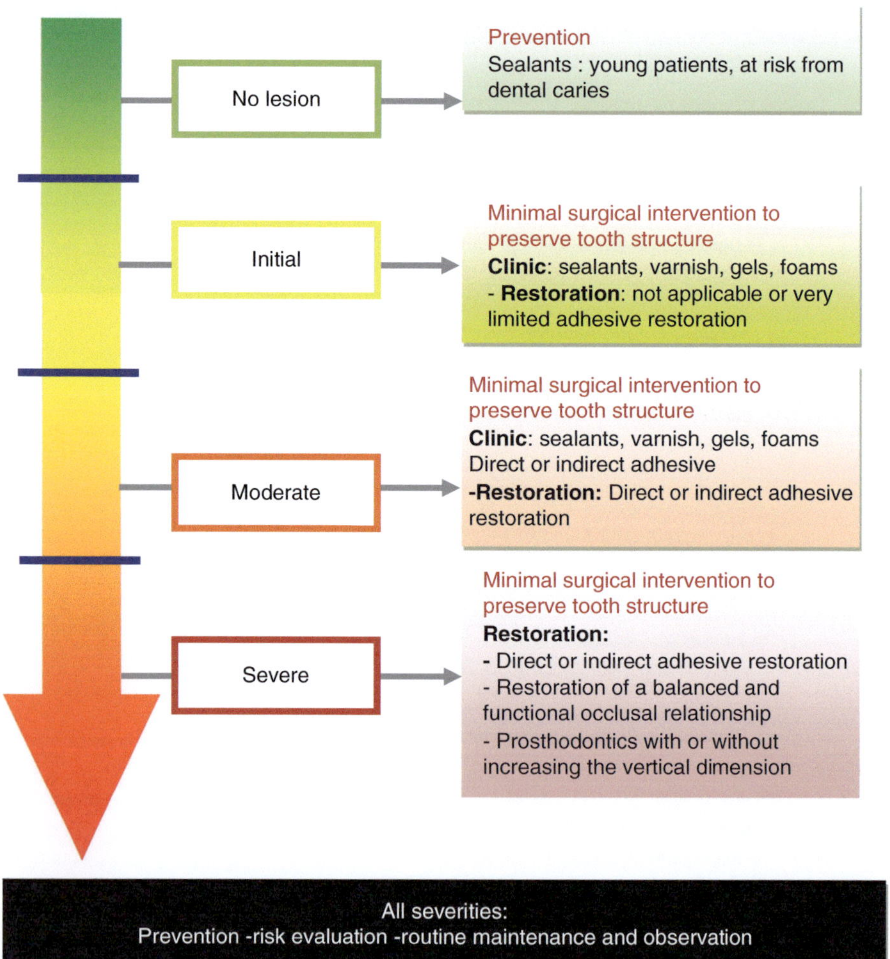

Fig. 20.5 A therapeutic classification for dental caries and erosion

References

American Academy of Pediatric Dentistry (2013) Policy on prevention of sports related orofacial injuries. Oral Health Policies 36:71–75

American Society for Testing and Materials (1986) Standard practice for care and use of mouthguards. Designation, Philadelphia, pp F697–F680. 323

Attin T, Weiss K, Becker K, Buchalla W, Wiegand A (2005) Impact of modified acidic soft drinks on enamel erosion. Oral Dis 11:7–12

Bartlett D, Ganss C, Lussi A (2008) Basic Erosive Wear Examination (BEWE): a new scoring system for scientific and clinical needs. Clin Oral Invest 12:65–68

Beauchamp J, Page W, Caufield J, Crall J, Donly K, Feigal R, Gooch B, Ismail A, Kohn W, Siegal M, Simonsen M (2008) Evidence-based clinical recommendations for the use of pit-and-fissure sealants: a report of the American Dental Association Council on Scientific Affairs. J Am Dent Assoc 139:257–268

Beslot-Neveu A, Courson F, Dorin N (2012) Physico-chemical approach to pit and fissure sealant infiltration and spreading mechanisms. Pediatr Dent 34:57–61

Carvalho TS, Colon P, Ganss C, Huysmans M, Lussi A, Schlueter N, Schmalz G, Shellis RP, Tveit AB, Wiegand A (2015) Consensus report of the European Federation of Conservative Dentistry: erosive tooth wear-diagnosis and management. Clin Oral Invest 19:1557–1561

Colon P, Lussi A (2014) Minimal intervention dentistry: part 5. Ultra-conservative approach to the treatment of erosive and abrasive lesions. Br Dent J 216:463–468

Featherstone JD (2000) The science and practice of caries prevention. J Am Dent Assoc 131:887–899

Ismail A, Tellez M, Pitts NB et al (2013) Caries management pathways preserve dental tissues and promote oral health. Community Dent Oral Epidemiol 41:12–40

Lamendin H (2004) Odontologie du Sport. Ed CdP, Paris

Lasfargues JJ, Colon P (2010) Odontologie Conservatrice Restauratrice: une approche médicale globale. Ed CdP, Paris

Liu BY, Lo ECM, Chu CH, Lin HC (2012) Randomized trial on fluorides and sealants for fissure caries prevention. J Dent Res 91:753–758

Murat M, İsmail Ş, Mustafa T (2007) Impacted teeth and mandibular fracture. Eur J Dent 1(1):18–20

21 The Treatment of Dental Trauma in Sport

21.1 Introduction

Dental emergencies resulting from traumatology in sport require quick thinking on the part of the dental practitioner. He must know how to deal efficiently with a vast array of potential accidents that affect the oral sphere.

A detailed medical anamnesis and evaluation of the accident's circumstances informs the dental surgeon of any potential infection, haemorrhagic or allergic risks during consequent dental treatment. Additionally, this information is required for medical certificates and referral to medical professionals.

The clinical examination must consider the patient globally, ensuring that vital functions are not affected. Both facial and oral hard and soft tissues must be inspected for fractures and lacerations. Tests of dental mobility, percussion and vitality are employed, to be confirmed by complimentary x-rays.

The therapeutic decision will depend on the lapse of time between the accident and consultation, the type and extent of trauma suffered and whether the teeth affected are classified as mature or immature in their stage of development.

21.2 A Concise Guide to the Treatment of Sports-Related Orofacial Trauma

The aim of the emergency treatment is to relieve pain, protect the patient from inflammation or the propagation of infection, to protect the vitality of teeth and to consolidate the traumatised elements.

Table 21.1 gives a concise overview of the different forms of dental traumatology commonly encountered in dental practice. The positive diagnosis of each lesion is detailed, as is the appropriate treatment in case of emergency. Focus is on permanent dentition, as athletes tend to take up sport during adolescence and upwards.

S.C. Budd, J.-C. Egea, *Sport and Oral Health*, DOI 10.1007/978-3-319-53423-7_21

Table 21.1 Principles of dental trauma care in sports dentistry

Dental trauma	Diagnosis	Treatment
Infraction 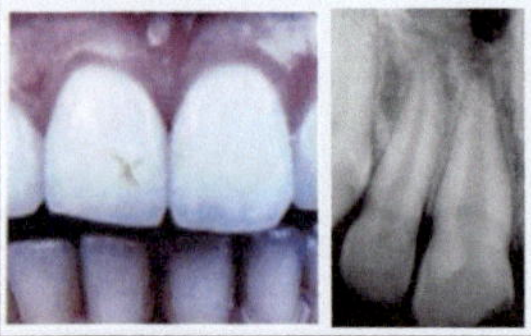	-Visible fracture line/crack on the tooth's surface	-N/A -Sealant
Enamel fracture 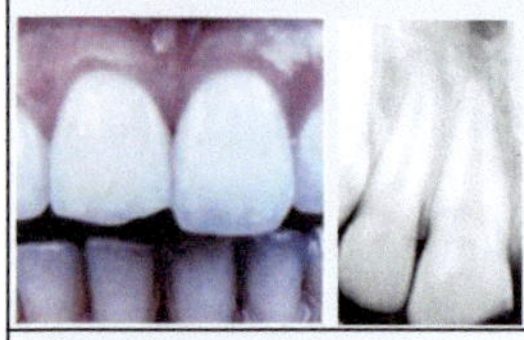	-Visible fracture of the enamel -Normal mobility	-Ameloplasty -Composite -X-ray controls
Enamel-dentin fracture 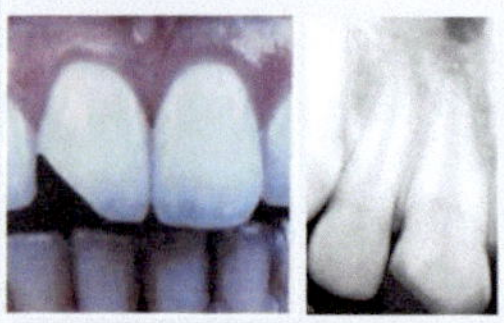	-Visible fracture of enamel-dentin, but pulp not exposed -Normal mobility	-Clean area -**$Ca(OH)_2$** capping if near pulp -Temporary CVI or -Definitive composite -X-ray: ensure root not fractured Dentin and pulp protection
Enamel-dentin pulp fracture 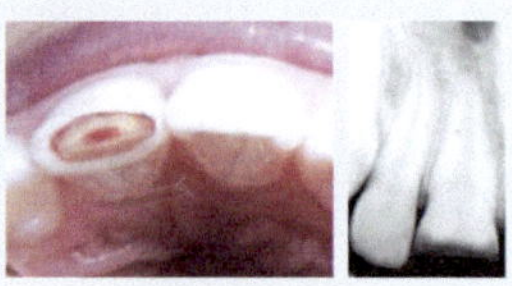	-Visible fracture of enamel-dentin with pulp exposure -Normal mobility -Vitality: normally +	-Clean area -**$Ca(OH)_2$** capping if near pulp -Temporary CVI or Definitive composite -X-ray: ensure root not fractured Dentin and pulp protection

Immature permanent teeth: focus on vitality preservation at all times

Table 21.1 (continued)

Dental trauma	Diagnosis	Treatment
Crown-root fracture 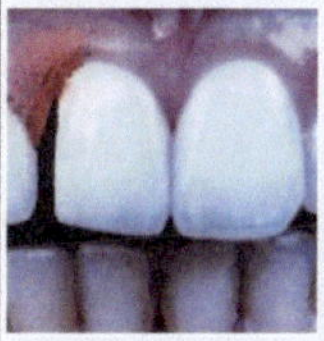 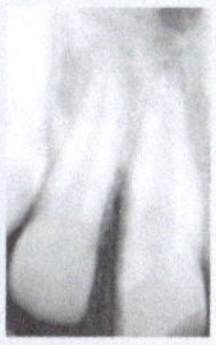	-Visible fracture of the enamel -Dentin-cementum crown fracture below gingival margin -Mobility of coronal fragment +++ -Vitality : normally + for apical segment	**Emergency**: possible stabilisation of loose segment to adjacent teeth **Definitive:** depends on fracture: -Remove fragment only & composite -Remove fragment & gingivectomy (envisage root canal treatment) -Orthodontic extrusion of apical fragment (& root canal treatment) -Surgical extrusion -Decoronation (then implantology) -Extraction
Crown-root fracture (with pulp involvement) 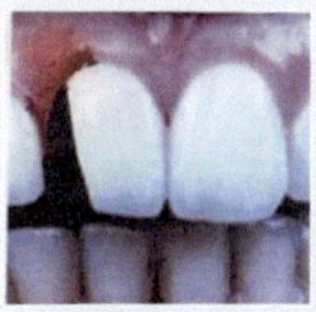 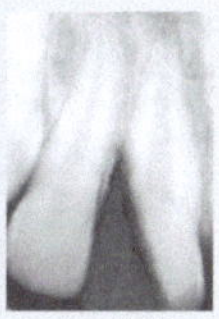	-Visible fracture of enamel-dentin-cementum with pulp exposure -Crown fracture below gingival margin -Mobility ++ of coronal fragment -Percussion: sensitive -Vitality: normally + for apical segment	**Emergency:** possible stabilisation of loose segment to adjacent teeth **Definitive:** depends on fracture: -Remove fragment only & composite -Remove fragment & gingivectomy (envisage root canal treatment) -Orthodontic extrusion of apical fragment (& root canal treatment) -Surgical extrusion -Decoronation (then implantology) -Extraction
Root fracture 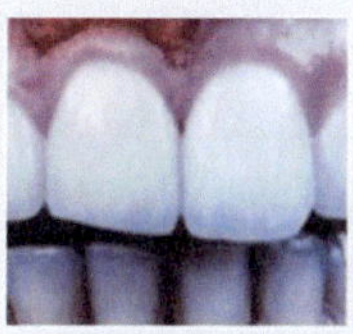 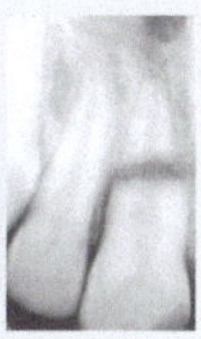	-Fracture of the Root: dentin-cementum & pulp -Crown fracture below gingival margin -Mobility possible: of coronal fragment -Possible decoloration of crown -Percussion: sensitive -Vitality: often - initially -Often visible on x-ray	**Emergency** -If not mobile: abstention -If mobile: Reposition the coronal fragment -Contention 4 weeks -Contention 3-4 months if 1/3 coronal section of the root **2nd Phase** -Monitor regularly pulp vitality, sensitivity and resorptions
Alveolar fracture 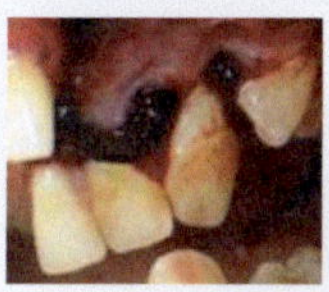 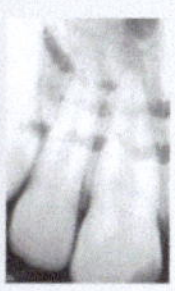	-Mobility of alveolar segment and teeth	**Emergency** -Reposition the fragment and dental structures involved -Contention 4 weeks **2nd Phase** -Monitor regularly pulp vitality, sensitivity and resorptions Antibiotics & anti inflammatories & antalgic & mouthwash

Table 21.1 (continued)

Dental trauma	Diagnosis	Treatment
Concussion 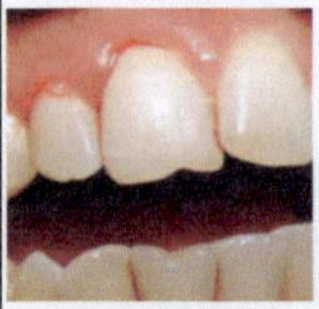 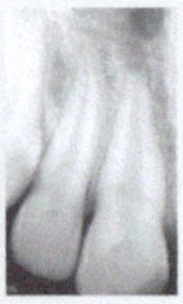	-No displacement or mobility -++ percussion -+ pulp sensitivity -No x-ray anomalies	-N/A -Monitor pulp sensitivity -Soft food & brush teeth after each meal -X-ray controls
Subluxation 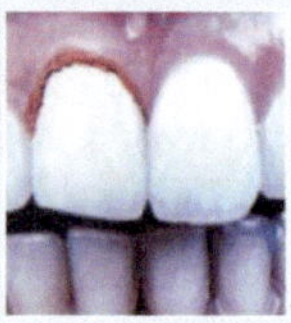 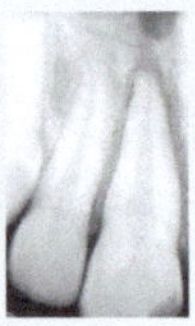	-Increased mobility -Not displaced -Percussion ++ -Vitality +/-	-N/A -Contention if needed - 2 weeks -Monitor pulp sensitivity -Soft food -X-raycontrols Antibiotics & anti inflammatories & antalgic & mouthwash
Lateral luxation 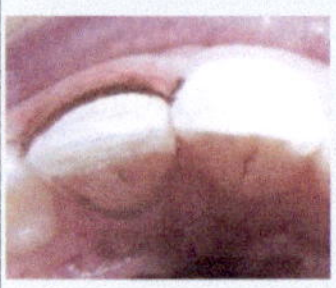 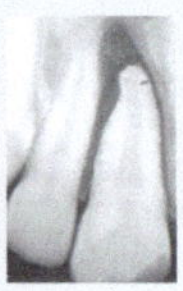	-Mobility +++ -Displaced: often palatal or lingual direction -Percussion +: metallic sound -Vitality +/- -Increased periapical ligament Space	-Anesthetic -Clean area with antibacterial product -Digital reposition or forceps (> 48h: orthodontic repositioning) -Contention: 4 weeks -X-ray controls ++ -Soft food & brush teeth after each meal Antibiotics & anti inflammatories & antalgic & mouthwash

Immature permanent teeth: focus on vitality preservation at all times

Table 21.1 (continued)

Dental trauma	Diagnosis	Treatment
Intrusion 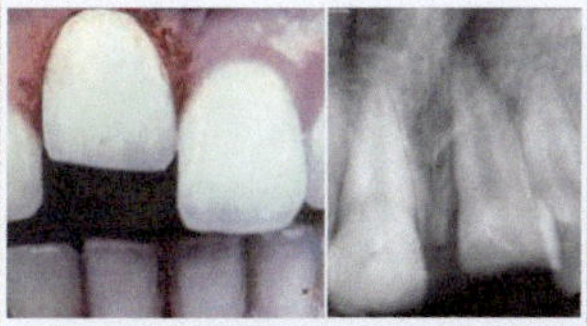	-Immobile -Displaced: axially into alveolar bone -Percussion +: metallic sound -Vitality - -Periapical ligament absence *-Immature tooth: revascularisation possible*	-Spontaneous eruption -Orthodontic repositioning -Surgical repositioning -Root canal treatment with **$Ca(OH)_2$** if unlikely pulp revascularisation -Controls ++ -Soft food & brush teeth after each meal Antibiotics & anti inflammatories & antalgic & mouthwash
Clinical case 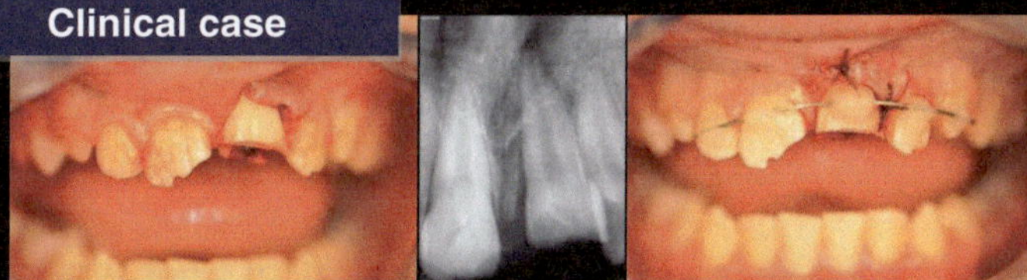		
Extrusion 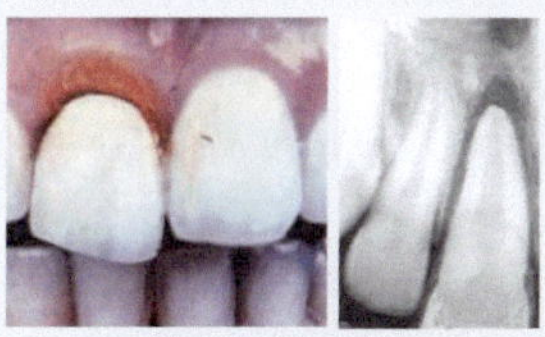	-Mobility +++ -Displaced: appears elongated -Percussion ++ -Vitality +/- -Increased periapical ligament space *-Immature tooth : revascularisation possible*	-Clean area -Digital reposition -Contention: 2 weeks -X-ray controls -Soft food & toothbrush after each meal
Clinical case 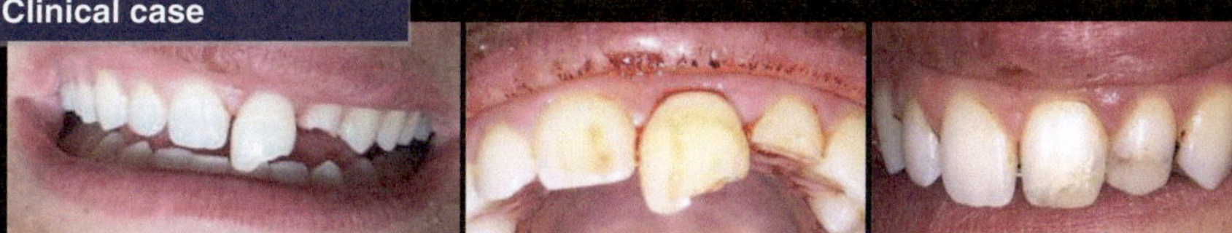		Antibiotics & anti inflammatories & antalgic & mouthwash
Courtesy of Dr Cedric Bourgeois		

Table 21.1 (continued)

Dental trauma	Diagnosis	Treatment
Avulsion 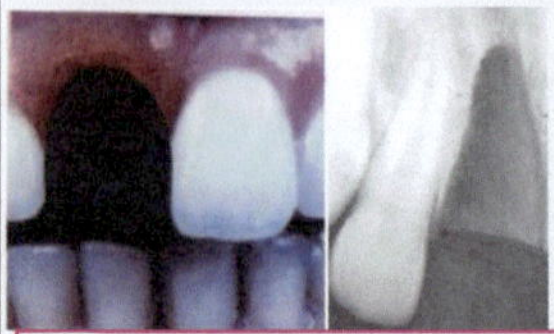 Antibiotics & anti inflammatories & antalgic & mouthwash		**Expulsion < 1 hour** **Emergency** -Rince alveole -Replace tooth -Supple contention **2nd Phase:** -Root canal treatment with **$Ca(OH)_2$** 7-10 days after *Immature tooth: revascularisation possible* -Controls +++ **Expulsion > 1 hour** **Emergency** -Rince alveole -Tooth in NaF solution: 20 mins -Replace tooth **2nd Phase:** -Root canal treatment with **$Ca(OH)_2$** 7-10 days afteror extra-oral root cnal treatment -Contention 4 weeks -Controls ++

Clinical case

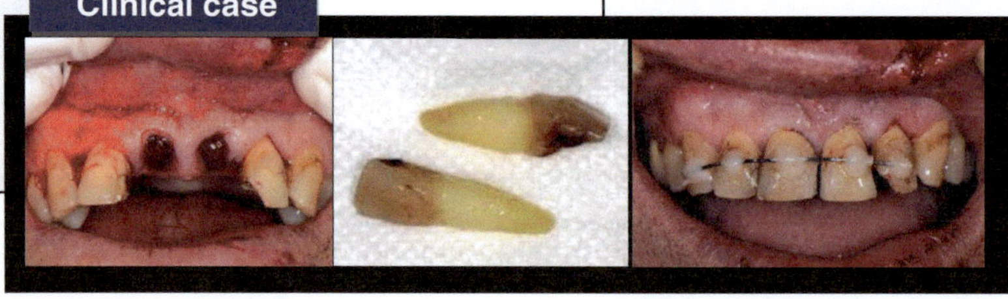

Doping, Prescription and Dentistry 22

22.1 Introduction

Doping in sport is controlled at different levels. National anti-doping bodies collaborate with the international World Anti-Doping Agency (WADA) which publishes an annual list of doping substances. A dental surgeon must protect an athlete's health, and the athlete, in turn, must admit all elements of his health and medication taken during a medical consultation.

The prescription of certain anti-inflammatories and antalgics in dentistry can pose a problem during an anti-doping control. However, an athlete may require a banned substance for justified health reasons. In this case, with help from his medical physician or dental surgeon, he may apply for a Therapeutic Use Exemption (TUE) from his national anti-doping agency. It is important to recognise that penal and disciplinary sanctions exist for both the athlete and the *health professional* who administered the prohibited molecule, in the event of substance abuse.

The World Anti-Doping Agency publishes an annual list of banned substances, applicable to both in and out of competition, which is easily accessible online. It is therefore important to keep up to date on any recent modifications or developments to avoid misconduct.

22.2 Prescription in Dental Practice

The main substances which could pose problems for the dental surgeon are *glucocorticoids* including prednisolone (Solupred®) and prednisone (Cortancyl®). Local applications, such as gels, creams and sprays are authorised. However, ingestion and injections are prohibited during competition.

Another molecule that may be problematic for athletes is codeine, an analgesic level II prescribed for severe dental pain. It is often associated with paracetamol. It is *not* prohibited. However, within certain individuals, its metabolism can give an abnormal result during an anti-doping test. Equally, a molecule to be taken into account is adrenaline (epinephrine). In dentistry, its association to local

S.C. Budd, J.-C. Egea, *Sport and Oral Health*, DOI 10.1007/978-3-319-53423-7_22

anaesthetic is *not* prohibited. However, it is on the list of banned substances if prescribed as a stimulant in general medicine. Precautions to take are therefore (a) to respect their posology and (b) to systematically signal their consumption during controls.

According to the World Anti-Doping Code, it is an athlete's duty to ensure that 'No *Prohibited Substance* enters his or her body and no *Prohibited Method* is utilized. *Athletes* are responsible for any *Prohibited Substance* and/or its *Metabolites* or *Markers* found to be present in any *Sample(s)* they provide and/or *Prohibited Method* detected from the *Sample*'.

22.3 Athletes Requiring Therapeutic Use Exemptions

Athletes with certain medical conditions which require the usage of prohibited substances in sport may demand their national anti-doping agency or international federation for a Therapeutic Use Exemption (TUE), which is based on international standards given by the WADA. The role of the TUE is therefore to permit an athlete with a medical condition to participate in his or her sport. A TUE is required for athletes of all levels, from the recreational participant to the international competitor. The dentist must supply the medical information required on the form, such as the molecule, its dosage and its mode of administration. Interestingly, the usage of glucocorticosteroids represented 36% of all TUEs (Vernec 2014).

Disciplinary and penal sanctions can exist for both athletes and health professionals. If we take the example of France, a dentist could be imprisoned for up to 5 years and receive a 75,000€ fine for ignoring their National Sports Code by purposely providing athletes with banned substances.

Figure 22.1 summarises the role of both the dental surgeon and athlete in the application for a Therapeutic Use Exemption from the US Anti-Doping Agency, which is obtainable from www.usada.org/substances/tue/apply/.

22.4 World Anti-Doping Code: Prohibited Substance List 2016

The World Anti-Doping Agency (WADA) annually publishes a list of substances and methods that are banned in the sporting world. It includes prohibited substances at all times (in and out of competition), prohibited substances during competition and prohibited substances in certain sports. It also includes prohibited methods.

The dentist must take care regarding his prescriptions. Furthermore, the dentist may also check that any other medications taken by the athlete for other medical reasons do not feature on this prohibited list.

Table 22.1 summarises the banned substances for 2016. Health professionals, coaches and athletes are advised to visit the WADA site on a regular basis to be up to date – https://www.wada-ama.org.

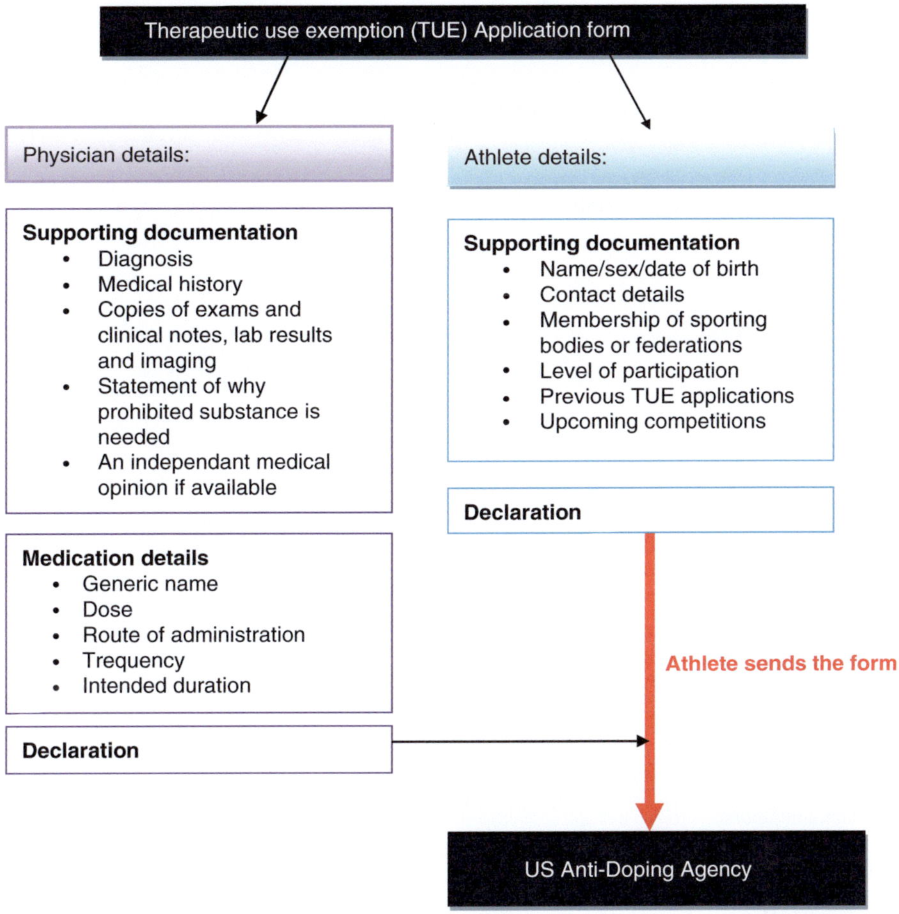

Fig. 22.1 Application for a Therapeutic Use Exemption (Source: www.usada.org/substances/tue/apply/)

Table 22.1 A summary of substances prohibited in sport

Prohibited substances at all times (in and out of competition)	Prohibited substances during competition	Prohibited substances in particular sports
1. Anabolic androgenic steroids (AAS) (a) Exogenous (b) Endogenous (c) Other anabolic agents	1. Stimulants 2. Narcotics 3. Cannabinoids 4. Glucocorticoids	1. Alcohol 2. Beta-blockers
2. Peptide hormones, growth factors and related substances	**PROHIBITED METHODS** • Manipulation of blood and blood components • Chemical and physicalmanipulation • Gene doping	
3. Beta-2 agonists		
4. Hormone and metabolic modulators		
5. Diuretics and masking agents		

Source: The World Anti-Doping Association (WADA) prohibited list 2016

22.5 Prohibited Substances at All Times (In and Out of Competition)

22.5.1 Anabolic Androgenic Steroids (AASs)

1a. Exogenous* AAS, including:
1-Androstenediol
1-Androstenedione
1-Testosterone
4-Hydroxytestosterone
19-Norandrostenedione
Bolandiol
Bolasterone
Boldenone
Boldione
Calusterone
Clostebol
Danazol
Dehydrochlormethyltestosterone
Desoxymethyltestosterone
Drostanolone
Ethylestrenol
Fluoxymesterone
Formebolone
Furazabol
Gestrinone
Mestanolone
Mesterolone
Methandienone
Methenolone
Methandriol
Methasterone
Methyldienolone
Methyl-1-testosterone
Methylnortestosterone
Methyltestosterone
Metribolone
Mibolerone
Nandrolone
Norboletone
Norclostebol
Norethandrolone
Oxabolone
Oxandrolone
Oxymesterone
Oxymetholone
Prostanozol
Quinbolone
Stanozolol
Stenbolone
Tetrahydrogestrinone
Trenbolone and other substances with a similar chemical structure or similar biological effect(s)

1b. Endogenous AAS when administered exogenously:**
Androstenediol
Androstenedione
Dihydrotestosterone
Prasterone
Testosterone and their metabolites and isomers, including but not limited to:
3β-Hydroxy-5α-androstan-17-one
5α-Androstane-3α,17α-diol
5α-Androstane-3α,17β-diol
5α-Androstane-3β,17α-diol
5α-Androstane-3β,17β-diol
5β-Androstane-3α,17β-diol
7α-Hydroxy-DHEA
7β-Hydroxy-DHEA
4-Androstenediol
5-Androstenedione
7-Keto-DHEA
19-Norandrosterone
19-Noretiocholanolone
Androst-4-ene-3α,17α-diol
Androst-4-ene-3α,17β-diol
Androst-4-ene-3β,17α-diol
Androst-5-ene-3α,17α-diol
Androst-5-ene-3α,17β-diol
Androst-5-ene-3β,17α-diol
Androsterone
Epi-dihydrotestosterone
Epitestosterone
Etiocholanolone

2. Other Anabolic Agents
Including, but not limited to: clenbuterol, selective androgen receptor modulators (SARMs, e.g. andarine and ostarine), tibolone, zeranol and zilpaterol

Key

'Exogenous' = a substance which is **not** ordinarily produced by the body naturally. 'Endogenous' = a substance which **is** ordinarily produced by the body naturally

22.5.2 Peptide Hormones, Growth Factors, Related Substances and Mimetics

1. **Erythropoietin receptor agonists**:
   1.1 Erythropoiesis-stimulating agents (ESAs) including, e.g. darbepoetin (dEPO); erythropoietin (EPO), EPO-Fc and EPO mimetic peptides (EMP), e.g. CNTO 530 and peginesatide; and methoxy polyethylene glycol-epoetin beta (CERA)
   1.2 Non-erythropoietic EPO-Receptor agonists, e.g. ARA-290, asialo EPO, carbamylated EPO
2. **Hypoxia-inducible factor (HIF) stabilisers**, e.g. cobalt and FG-4592, and HIF activators, e.g. argon and xenon
3. **Chorionic gonadotrophin (CG) and luteinising hormone (LH)** and their releasing factors, e.g. buserelin, gonadorelin and leuprorelin, in males
4. **Corticotrophins and their releasing factors**, e.g. corticorelin
5. **Growth hormone (GH)** and its releasing factors including:
   Growth hormone-releasing hormone (GHRH) and its analogues, e.g. CJC-1295, sermorelin and tesamorelin
   Growth hormone secretagogues (GHS), e.g. ghrelin and ghrelin mimetics, e.g. anamorelin and ipamorelin
   GH-releasing peptides (GHRPs), e.g. alexamorelin, GHRP-6, hexarelin and pralmorelin (GHRP-2)

Additional prohibited growth factors:

Fibroblast growth factors (FGFs)
Hepatocyte growth factor (HGF)
Insulin-like growth factor-1 (IGF-1) and its analogues
Mechano growth factors (MGFs)
Platelet-derived growth factor (PDGF)
Vascular endothelial growth factor (VEGF) and any other growth factors affecting muscle, tendon or ligament protein synthesis/degradation, vascularisation, energy utilisation, regenerative capacity or fibre-type switching

22.5.3 Beta-2 Agonists

All beta-2 agonists, including all optical isomers, e.g. d- and l- where relevant, are prohibited.

Except:

- Inhaled salbutamol (maximum 1600 micrograms over 24 h)
- Inhaled formoterol (maximum delivered dose 54 micrograms over 24 h)
- Inhaled salmeterol in accordance with the manufacturers' recommended therapeutic regimen

The presence in urine of salbutamol in excess of 1000 ng/mL or formoterol in excess of 40 ng/mL is presumed not to be an intended therapeutic use of the substance and will be considered as an adverse analytical finding (AAF) unless the athlete proves, through a controlled pharmacokinetic study, that the abnormal result was the consequence of the use of the therapeutic inhaled dose up to the maximum indicated above.

22.5.4 Hormone and Metabolic Modulators

1. **Aromatase inhibitors including, but not limited to**:
   4-Androstene-3,6,17-trione (6-oxo)
   Aminoglutethimide
   Anastrozole
   Androsta-1,4,6-triene-3,17-dione (androstatrienedione)
   Exemestane
   Formestane
   Letrozole
   Testolactone
2. **Selective estrogen receptor modulators (SERMs) including, but not limited to**:
   Raloxifene
   Tamoxifen
   Toremifene
3. **Other anti-estrogenic substances including, but not limited to**:
   Clomiphene
   Cyclofenil
   Fulvestrant
4. **Agents modifying myostatin function(s) including, but not limited, to myostatin inhibitors**
5. **Metabolic modulators**
   5.1 Activators of the AMP-activated protein kinase (AMPK), e.g. AICAR, and peroxisome proliferator-activated receptor δ (PPARδ) agonists, e.g. GW 1516

5.2 Insulins and insulin mimetics
5.3 Meldonium
5.4 Trimetazidine

22.5.5 Diuretics and Masking Agents

Including, but not limited to:

Desmopressin, probenecid, plasma expanders, e.g. glycerol and intravenous administration of albumin, dextran, hydroxyethyl starch and mannitol

Acetazolamide; amiloride; bumetanide; canrenone; chlortalidone; etacrynic acid; furosemide; indapamide; metolazone; spironolactone; thiazides, e.g. bendroflumethiazide, chlorothiazide and hydrochlorothiazide; triamterene and vaptans, e.g. tolvaptan

Except: drospirenone, pamabrom and ophthalmic use of carbonic anhydrase inhibitors (e.g. dorzolamide, brinzolamide)

Local administration of felypressin in dental anaesthesia

The detection in an athlete's sample at all times or in competition, as applicable, of any quantity of the following substances subject to threshold limits, formoterol, salbutamol, cathine, ephedrine, methylephedrine and pseudoephedrine, in conjunction with a diuretic or masking agent, will be considered as an adverse analytical finding unless the athlete has an approved **TUE** for that substance in addition to the one granted for the diuretic or masking agent.

22.6 Prohibited in Competition Only

22.6.1 Stimulants

All stimulants, including all optical isomers, e.g. d- and l- where relevant, are prohibited.

(a): **Non-specified stimulants**

Adrafinil
Amfepramone
Amphetamine
Amphetaminil
Amiphenazole
Benfluorex
Benzylpiperazine
Bromantan
Clobenzorex
Cocaine
Cropropamide
Crotetamide
Fencamine
Fenethylline
Fenfluramine
Fenproporex
Fonturacetam [4-phenylpiracetam (carphedon)]
Furfenorex
Mefenorex
Mephentermine
Mesocarb
Methamphetamine (d-)
p-Methylamphetamine
Modafinil
Norfenfluramine
Phendimetrazine
Phentermine
Prenylamine
Prolintane

(b): Specified stimulants
Including, but not limited to:
Benzphetamine
Cathine**
Cathinone and its analogues, e.g. mephedrone, methedrone and α- pyrrolidinovalerophenone
Dimethylamphetamine
Ephedrine***
Epinephrine**** (adrenaline)
Etamivan
Etilamfetamine
Etilefrine
Famprofazone
Fenbutrazate
Fencamfamin
Heptaminol
Hydroxyamphetamine (parahydroxyamphetamine)
Isometheptene
Levomethamphetamine
Meclofenoxate
Methylenedioxymethamphetamine
Methylephedrine***
Methylhexanamine (dimethylpentylamine)
Methylphenidate
Nikethamide
Norfenefrine
Octopamine
Oxilofrine (methylsynephrine)
Pemoline
Pentetrazol
Phenethylamine and its derivatives
Phenmetrazine
Phenpromethamine
Propylhexedrine
Pseudoephedrine*****
Selegiline
Sibutramine
Strychnine
Tenamfetamine (methylenedioxyamphetamine)
Tuaminoheptane and other substances with a similar chemical structure or similar biological effect(s)

Except:
- Clonidine
- Imidazole derivatives for topical/ophthalmic use and those stimulants included in the 2016 Monitoring Program*

* Bupropion, caffeine, nicotine, phenylephrine, phenylpropanolamine, pipradrol and synephrine: these substances are included in the 2016 Monitoring Program and are not considered prohibited substances.
** Cathine: prohibited when its concentration in urine is greater than 5 micrograms per millilitre.
*** Ephedrine and methylephedrine: prohibited when the concentration of either in urine is greater than 10 micrograms per millilitre.
**** Epinephrine (adrenaline): not prohibited in local administration, e.g. nasal and ophthalmologic, or co-administration with local anaesthetic agents.
***** Pseudoephedrine: prohibited when its concentration in urine is greater than 150 micrograms per millilitre.

22.6.2 Narcotics

Prohibited:

Buprenorphine
Dextromoramide
Diamorphine (heroin)
Fentanyl and its derivatives
Hydromorphone
Methadone
Morphine
Oxycodone
Oxymorphone
Pentazocine
Pethidine

22.6.3 Cannabinoids

Prohibited:

- Natural, e.g. cannabis, hashish and marijuana, or synthetic Δ9-tetrahydrocannabinol (THC)
- Cannabimimetics, e.g. 'spice', JWH-018, JWH-073, HU-210

22.6.4 Glucocorticoids

All glucocorticoids are prohibited when administered by oral, intravenous, intramuscular or rectal routes.

22.7 Substances Prohibited in *Particular Sports*

22.7.1 Alcohol

Alcohol (ethanol) is prohibited in competition only, in the following sports. Detection will be conducted by analysis of breath and/or blood. The doping violation threshold is equivalent to a blood alcohol concentration of 0.10 g/L:

- Air sports (FAI)
- Automobile (FIA)
- Archery (WA)
- Powerboating (UIM)

22.7.2 Beta-Blockers

Beta-blockers are prohibited in competition only, in the following sports, and also prohibited

Out of competition where indicated:

- Archery (WA)*
- Automobile (FIA)
- Billiards (all disciplines) (WCBS)
- Darts (WDF)
- Golf (IGF)
- Shooting (ISSF, IPC)*
- Skiing/snowboarding (FIS) in ski jumping, freestyle aerials/halfpipe and snowboard halfpipe/big air
- Underwater sports (CMAS) in constant weight apnoea with or without fins, dynamic apnoea with and without fins, free immersion apnoea, jump blue apnoea, spearfishing, static apnoea, target shooting and variable weight apnoea

*Also prohibited out of competition

Including, but not limited to:

Acebutolol
Alprenolol
Atenolol
Betaxolol
Bisoprolol
Bunolol
Carteolol
Carvedilol
Celiprolol
Esmolol
Labetalol
Levobunolol
Metipranolol
Metoprolol
Nadolol
Oxprenolol
Pindolol
Propranolol
Sotalol
Timolol

References

Vernec A. Therapeutic Use Exemption : Principles and Practice. WADA TUE Symposium, Paris. 2014. https://www.wada-ama.org/sites/default/files/resources/files/01-vernecalan-tue_symposium_paris_vernec_october_23_2014.pdf. Accessed 25 Nov 2016

World Anti-Doping Agency. World Anti Doping Code Article 2.2.1. https://www.wada-ama.org/en/resources/the-code/world-anti-doping-code (2016). Accessed 26 Nov 2016

Conclusion 23

In recent years, thousands of individuals have turned to sport in order to get into shape, relieve stress and improve their physical health. Such popularity has been actively encouraged by governmental health promotion schemes and the organisation of numerous sporting events, open to athletes of all levels, not just the elite.

Paradoxically, in the pursuit of a healthier lifestyle and peak physical performance, oral health may be compromised. Behavioural, psychological and physiological risk factors predispose athletes to a vast array of undesirable oral consequences. The effects are multiple and affect the athlete on different levels. Constituents of the oral cavity, such as hard dental surfaces, periodontal structures and saliva flow rate, may be adversely affected. Furthermore, dental pain, the systemic spread of oral infection, traumatology and perturbations of dental occlusion affect an athlete's physical health, his psychological wellbeing and athletic performance.

Many athletes are currently unaware of the intricate relationship between oral health and sport, and the role of the dental practitioner has been overlooked. The dental surgeon is an integral actor of an athlete's support network, alongside a variety of health professionals including physiotherapists, osteopaths and physicians.

To increase the awareness amongst professionals and athletes, oral health promotion and disease prevention strategies must be reinforced within medical, paramedical and educational sectors. But equally, the dental surgeon must also be able to correlate certain sports medical information to the field of dentistry.

Athletes require a specific monitoring of their oral health. The practitioner must inform and educate and evaluate their patient's individual fragility as from the first consultation. The key to sustainable oral health is prevention and regular medical supervision, as the slightest interference to good oral health can undo months of sporting preparation.

A well-adapted multidisciplinary treatment plan will avoid such repercussions and help the athlete achieve their desired optimal condition of physical, psychological and social wellbeing.

S.C. Budd, J.-C. Egea, *Sport and Oral Health*, DOI 10.1007/978-3-319-53423-7_23

Table of Illustrations

Figures

S.C. Budd, J.-C. Egea, *Sport and Oral Health*, DOI 10.1007/978-3-319-53423-7

Tables

Index

S.C. Budd, J.-C. Egea, *Sport and Oral Health*, DOI 10.1007/978-3-319-53423-7

MIX
Papier aus verantwortungsvollen Quellen
Paper from responsible sources
FSC® C105338

If you have any concerns about our products,
you can contact us on
ProductSafety@springernature.com

In case Publisher is established outside the EU,
the EU authorized representative is:
Springer Nature Customer Service Center GmbH
Europaplatz 3, 69115 Heidelberg, Germany

Printed by Libri Plureos GmbH
in Hamburg, Germany